Compendium of Surface Microscopic and Dermoscopic Features

Volker Paech
Hans Schulz
Zsolt Argenyi
Thilo Gambichler
Peter Altmeyer

Volker Paech · Hans Schulz · Zsolt Argenyi
Thilo Gambichler · Peter Altmeyer

Compendium of Surface Microscopic and Dermoscopic Features

With 195 Figures and 17 Tables

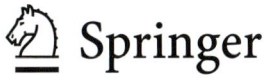 Springer

Dr. Volker Paech
Priv.-Doz. Dr. Thilo Gambichler
Prof. Dr. Peter Altmeyer
Universität Bochum
Klinik für Dermatologie und Allergologie
St. Josef Hospital
Gudrunstr. 56
44791 Bochum
Germany

Dr. Hans Schulz
Im Alten Dorf 8
59192 Bergkamen
Germany

Prof. Zsolt Argenyi, MD
University of Washington
Medical Center
Dermatopathology
1959 N.E. Pacific 356100
Seattle, WA 98195-6100
USA

ISBN 978-3-540-78972-7   e-ISBN 978-3-540-78973-4

DOI 10.1007/978-3-540-78973-4

Library of Congress Control Number: 2008924904

Cover design: Frido Steinen-Broo, eStudio Calamar, Spain
Production & Typesetting: le-tex publishing services oHG, Leipzig, Germany

Printed on acid-free paper

9 8 7 6 5 4 3 2 1

springer.com

Preface

The main focus of this book is to provide a comprehensive, current, and accurate lexicon to expand and clarify the meaning of surface microscopic and dermoscopic terminology including a broad range of both melanocytic and non-melanocytic skin lesions. In accordance with Stolz et al. (2002) we use the term skin "surface microscopy" as a general one, and prefer "dermoscopy" for examination of the skin with 10-fold magnification. The rapid advance of new technological approaches in dermatologic diagnosis, i.e., computer-aided surface microscopy and teledermoscopy via the Internet, facilitates consultation and exchange of information between physicians of different disciplines. As a result of these advances, surface microscopy and dermoscopy now have a worldwide acceptance as an important in vivo diagnostic step between the macroscopic–clinical and the subsequent microscopic–histological evaluation. The anatomical structures seen using this novel technique create a new terminology and a set of dermoscopic criteria. We believe the contents of this book will help dermatologists, histopathologists and physicians of other medical specialties in determining whether the lesion needs to be biopsied, excised, or can be left along for observation only. The daily challenge physicians face when evaluating skin lesions requires immediate access to the current dermoscopic nomenclature and definition. In the past, many different and sometimes confusing terms have been used in designating the surface microscopic features.

However, the generally accepted nomenclature and the definitions used in this book are based on the authors' observations and the following publications:

- Marghoob AA, Braun RP, Kopf AW (2005) Atlas of dermoscopy. Taylor & Francis, London New York

- Menzies SW, Crotty KA, Ingvar C, McCarthy WH (2003) An Atlas of surface microscopy of pigmented skin lesions: dermoscopy. McGraw-Hill Book Company, Sydney New York
- Stolz W, Braun-Falco O, Bilek P, Landthaler M, Burgdorf WHC, Cognetta AB (2002) Color atlas of dermatoscopy. Blackwell, Berlin

The main histopathologic terms and definitions applied in this book are adapted from the following publications:

- Ackerman AB, Maize JC (1987) Pigmented lesions of the skin. Lea & Febiger, Philadelphia
- Ackerman AB (1990) A dermatopathologist's guide to melanocytic nevi and malignant melanomas for surgeons. In: Conley J (ed) Melanoma of the head and neck. Thieme, Stuttgart New York, pp 9–33
- Braun-Falco O, Plewig G, Wolff HH, Winkelmann RK (1991) Dermatology. Springer, Berlin Heidelberg New York
- Hölzle E, Kind P, Plewig G, Burgdorf W (1993) Malignant melanoma. Diagnosis and differential diagnosis. Schattauer, Stuttgart New York

All surface microscopy photographs presented here were achieved using a microDerm videodermatoscopic system and an Olympus macrophotographic unit (OM-4Ti). Red bars integrated in the figures are at intervals of 1 mm. The fine black circle lines are spaced in 0.16- or 0.4-mm intervals.

Volker Paech
Hans Schulz
Zsolt Argenyi
Thilo Gambichler
Peter Altmeyer

Introduction

The history of skin surface microscopy dates back to the German dermatologist Johann Saphier (1920) who had published a series of communications using a new diagnostic apparatus composed of a binocular microscope with an integrated source of light for the examination of the skin. He had used this apparatus in different indications and presented some very interesting morphological observations concerning the anatomical structures of the skin. Thirty years later, Leon Goldman (1951) published a series of articles on new instruments to be used in so-called "dermoscopy" techniques. Goldman was the first dermatologist who used this technique in the assessment of pigmented lesions. MacKie et al. (1971) described the use of a dermoscope for the pre-surgical assessment of pigmented lesions. Since then, researchers all over the world started to work in the field of dermoscopy. This new approach in the diagnosis of pigmented lesions identified a great number of structures that are invisible on clinical examination. Today, dermoscopy is a routine technique predominantly used in European countries and recognized by many others.

Dermoscopy is a non-invasive, diagnostic imaging technique which allows the visualization of subtle clinical features of the skin surface and its underlying structures normally not visible to the unaided eye. The technique has also been referred to as epiluminescence microscopy, episcopy or dermatoscopy. The basic principle of dermoscopy is transillumination of the lesion and examining it with adequate magnification to visualize subtle features. The incident light on skin undergoes reflection, refraction, diffraction and absorption. These phenomena are influenced by the physical properties of the skin. Most of the incident light on the dry and scaly skin is reflected, but the smooth, well-hydrated or oily skin allows most of the light to pass through it, reaching the deeper dermis. This principle has been applied to improve the visibility of subsurface skin structures by employing contact media fluids over the lesions to improve the translucency of the skin. Various contact fluids have been tried such as oils (e.g., olive oil), water, antiseptic solutions, and glycerin. Water or antiseptic solutions can evaporate quickly and hence are less preferred than oils. Frequently, liquid paraffin is used, which is inexpensive, safe and easily available, with good results. Glass has a refractive index very similar to that of skin and hence when placed over oil-applied skin, further enhances transillumination of the lesion. The essential components of a dermoscope are 1) an achromatic lens, 2) an integrated illuminating system, and 3) a power supply. The achromatic lenses used for dermoscopy usually provide 10-fold magnification. The halogen lamps oriented at an angle of 20° are placed within the handheld piece of the dermoscope. The color contrasts of lesions are altered by the yellow light of halogen lamps. Some dermoscopes are equipped with light emitting diodes providing high intensity white light and consume 70% less power than halogen lamps. Illumination can be altered by turning off a set of light emitting diodes. They are also designed to emit lights of different colors for better visualization of the skin as penetration of the skin by light is proportional to the wavelength of light. Handheld instruments are usually powered by batteries housed in the instrument handles such as lithium ion, rechargeable lithium, or AA batteries. Additional facilities in some of the dermoscopes are an inbuilt photography system, either an attachable conventional or digital camera or an inbuilt camera, and supporting software, for the capture, storage, retrieval and even diagnostic software for interpretation the of images.

Principally, dermoscopic devices can be classified as simple instruments without image capturing facility (e.g, DELTA 20®, Mini 3000 Dermatoscope®), instruments with image capturing facility (e.g., Fotoadapter SLR für Delta 20®), and instruments with image capturing facility and analytical capability such as DermoGenius MoleMap®, Fotofinder dermoscope®, Molemax II®, and microDERM®. Dermoscopes with image capturing diagnostic features are increasingly used to improve dermoscopes for clinical diagnosis, preoperative assessment, and follow-up of pigmented lesions. Archived images of the patient can be compared with the new ones for assessing any subtle changes, otherwise not appreciable for the convential examination. Artificial neural network algorithms help to judge whether a melanocytic nevus is benign. Computer-based analysis of pigmented skin lesions is potentially suitable for both pre-screening of patients performed by non-experienced operators (e.g., nurses) and for clinicians' decision-making in the evaluation of pigmented lesions. Furthermore, computerized analysis of dermoscopy images may serve as an additional tool to improve follow-ups of patients, in particular those with multiple atypical nevi. Although dermoscopes are largely used for the study of pigmented skin lesions, such as melanocytic nevi and melanoma, they can also be used to aid diagnosing other conditions, including psoriasis, lichen planus, dermatofibroma, Darier's disease, cicatricial alopecia, seborrhoeic keratosis, scabies, and urticarial vasculitis. Since advanced cutaneous melanoma is still considered incurable, early detection by means of accurate screening is an important step toward reducing mortality. Usually, the screening tests are simple and only require a brief skin examination by an experienced investigator. The ABCDE rule is one of the most widely used methods for evaluating pigmented skin lesions with the naked eye. For the many difficult or borderline pigmented skin lesions, however, diagnostic accuracy is only slightly above 60% even in specialized centers. Several studies have shown that dermoscopy improves diagnostic accuracy by 20% to 30% with respect to simple clinical observation, especially by an expert dermatologist. Numerous studies in this field have cumulated a body of specific dermoscopic criteria, paving the way for a new semiology that provides the analysis of patterns, colors, intensities of pigmentation, configuration, regularity, and margin and surface characteristics. Well-defined dermoscopy methods for the diagnosis of melanoma that are even suitable for inexperienced clinicians have been developed. This allows formal training in dermoscopy that is necessary to improve diagnostic accuracy.

With the advent of computers, dermoscopic equipment has become easier and more economical to use. Digital dermatoscopy is increasingly used in clinical practice. The digital dermatoscopic systems available today provide images of excellent quality, similar to the quality of analogue photographs. They all offer the possibility of storing dermatoscopic images and patient data. Another interesting domain that is being developed is teledermoscopy. At the onset of digital dermatoscopy, teledermoscopy was used by experts who wished to submit their difficult or very interesting cases. The rapid development of new media services and the Internet technology will probably have great influence, because the infrastructure has become available for the majority of users. Therefore teledermoscopy may be utilized without prior extensive knowledge in computing. Apart from dermoscopy, there are other skin imaging techniques that are currently being evaluated in the field of skin cancer diagnosis in vivo. High-frequency ultrasound operating in the range of 20 MHz usually offers a relatively high depth of penetration, while resolution remains insufficient to study skin morphology in detail. However, ultrasound transducers with a center frequency of around 100 MHz are expected to be used for future diagnostic tissue characterization because of their relatively high lateral resolution. The latter technique may be particularly useful for the preoperative assessment of melanoma thickness. Optical coherence tomography, a method for imaging the structure of biological tissue in vivo with micron resolution, has been recognized as a promising tool for the diagnosis of pathological changes in various biological tissues. Depending on the scattering properties of tissue and some accepted loss in resolution, a penetration depth of about 500–1000 μm can be achieved with optical coherence tomography. New systems with ultra-high resolution of about 1 μm have recently been developed, however, lateral resolution of 10–15 μm is more typical. Optical coherence tomography is capable to present cross-sectional high resolution images of structures below the tissue surface in analogy to histology. It has been shown that optical coherence tomography allows for the differentiation of benign nevi from malignant melanoma on the basis of visual analysis of opticl coherence tomography images. Confocal laser scanning microscopy is currently the most challenging non-invasive imaging technique for skin cancer diagnosis in vivo, since it is capable to enable skin imaging with a lateral resolution of less than 1 μm. Thus, confocal laser scanning microscopy makes it possible to study the skin on the cellular and subcellular level in vivo. Nevertheless, in contrast to optical coherence tomography and high-frequency ultrasound, confocal laser scanning microscopy provides horizontal sections and is encumbered by the small field of examination, the mirror-based design, and limited depths of imaging of about 250 μm. There is now a wealth of evidence suggesting that confocal laser scanning microscopy may be useful to non-invasively discriminate benign nevi and malignant melanoma in vivo. Spectrophotometric intracutaneous analysis (SIAscopy) is a light-based imaging system capable of producing rapid images of melanin, blood and collagen of the skin. The first clinical trial with SIAscopy has yielded very promising results with new information useful to the clinician diagnosing pigmented skin lesions. The implementation of the aforementioned techniques in conjunction with dermoscopy could significantly improve the in-vivo diagnosis of skin lesions, and therefore promise a great diagnostic advance in the future.

References

11; 14; 19; 43; 65; 84; 100; 101; 106; 115; 119; 120; 164; 168; 192; 195; 199; 201; 216; 224; 243; 269

Contents

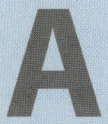

ABCD Rule of Dermoscopy

Definition

The ABCD rule of dermoscopy (Table 1) was the first method of the so-called melanoma algorithms in dermoscopy. With a scoring system (total dermoscopy score, TDS), a grading of pigmented lesions is possible with respect to their malignant potential. The TDS is used to classify the lesion as benign (TDS < 4.75), suspicious (TDS < 4.75–5.45), or malignant (TDS > 5.45).

References

42; 95; 123; 146; 165; 219; 266; 270; 293; 295; 297

ABC Point List of Dermoscopy

Definition

The ABC point list of dermoscopy (Table 2) is a point-list algorithm to discriminate benign melanocytic lesions from cutaneous melanoma. It is based on statistical analysis. A lesion should be considered a malignant lesion if the score is four points or higher.

References

45; 46; 95; 123; 219; 266

◘ Table 1 The ABCD rule of dermoscopy. (Modified from Semmelmayer et al. 2005)

	Score
Asymmetry	0–2
In zero, one or two axes; color, texture, and shape	
Border	0–8
Abrupt cut-off of pigment pattern in 0–8 segments	
Color	1–6
Presence of up to six colors (white, red, light brown, dark brown, blue-gray, black)	
Differential structures	1–5
Presence of network, structureless areas, dots, globules, and streaks	

◘ Table 2 The ABC point list of dermoscopy. (Modified from Blum et al. 2003)

Feature	Description	Point
Asymmetry	Asymmetry of shape in at least one axis	1
(A)symmetry	Asymmetry of structures in at least one axis	1
Border	Abrupt border cut-off (> 25% of the lesion)	1
Color	Three or more colors (white, red, light brown, dark brown, blue-gray, black	1
Differential structures	Three or more: network, homogeneous areas (> 10% of total surface); streaks (more than two); globules (more than two); black/brown dots (more than two)	1
Evolution	History of change in last 3 months	+1
	No/uncertain information	0
	No history of change reported	−1

Abrupt Cut-off of the Trabeculae

Synonyms
Synonyms for abrupt cut-off of the trabeculae are abrupt edge and abrupt pigment breaks in the trabeculae.

Definition
Melanocytic lesion with sharp breaks of pigmentation within the network pattern. That may occur in some trabeculae in the center of the lesion or at the peripheral network without a smooth transition into the normal skin (abrupt edge).

Occurrence
An abrupt edge in any part of the lesion suggests malignant melanoma. Abrupt cut-offs in the trabeculae may suggest dysplastic nevus.

References
189; 263

Abrupt Edge

▶ Abrupt cut-off of the trabeculae.

Abrupt Pigment Breaks in the Trabeculae

▶ Abrupt cut-off of the trabeculae.

Acantholysis

Definition
Acantholysis is a loss of cell-to-cell continuity or separation of individual epidermal keratinocytes from their neighbor, in conditions such as Darier's disease, actinic keratosis, herpes infection, and pemphigus vulgaris. Acantholytic vesicles often begin in the suprabasal layer with initial crevice-shaped vesicles. In surface microscopy this causes the phenomenon of so-called naked papillae since the capillary loops within the dermal papillae become visible.

Acanthoma

Definition
Acanthoma is a tumor formed by proliferation of epithelial squamous cells, e.g., keratoacanthoma (hairpin-like-shaped blood vessels) and melanoacanthoma.

Acanthosis

Definition
An increase in the thickness of the stratum spinosum (spinous cell layer) of the epidermis. Under surface microscopy this may appear as an opaque hue overlying the dermal papillae. The color in acanthotic epidermis ranges from opaque whitish-yellow to yellowish-brownish or gray-brownish.

Accessory Nipple

▶ Supernumerary nipple.

Acne Rosacea

▶ Corticosteroid side effects.

Acrolentiginous Melanoma

Synonym
The synonym for acrolentiginous melanoma is acral lentiginous melanoma (ALM).

Definition
An irregularly demarcated malignant melanocytic lesion, characteristically developing from clinical lentigo-type lesions, presenting at acral location (palms, soles, nail bed, and on the genitalia) or on mucous membranes (Fig. 1).

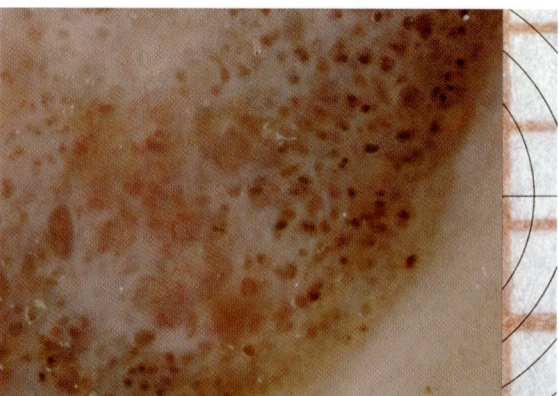

◘ **Fig. 1** Acrolentiginous melanoma on the sole (Clark level V, Breslow thickness 3.1 mm) shows irregular band-like pigmentations with dots and globules (crista dotted pattern) on the surface ridges

Surface Microscopy

In early phases of ALM the parallel ridge pattern (PRP) shows band-like pigmentation with color variegation from tan to black on the ridges of the surface skin markings. Occasionally, ALM can be amelanotic. PRP, i.e., the macular in-situ component, is highly suggestive in detecting early and invasive acrolentiginous melanoma with a sensitivity of 86% and a specificity of 99%. A characteristic feature in more advanced lesions is an irregular diffuse pigmentation with variable shades (multicomponent pigmentation). Sulci of the skin markings are often spared from pigmentation, creating the appearance of parallel furrow pattern, lattice-like pattern, fibrillar pattern, and crista dotted pattern, which are sometimes seen within the macular portions of ALM. Additional features are as follows: peripheral dots/globules, irregularly distributed brown or black globules, streaks, saccular pattern, abrupt edge, blue-white veil, and a peppering of multiple gray dots. In earlier stages subungual melanoma present as a tan pigmented band of the nail plate, often composed of numerous smaller sub-bands varying in color and width. Nevertheless, some of the subungual tumors are amelanotic. Longitudinal melanonychia striata, with hyponychial pigmentation showing the PRP, especially the latter, are referred to as Hutchinson's sign (i.e., extension of pigmentation to periungual skin), and is highly suspicious for ALM. Nail dystrophy, sometimes in the absence of pigmentation, indicates the onset of invasion. On mucous membranes the tumors are usually macular presenting blue-gray or brown hazy extensions in addition with perivascular aggregations of slate-gray granules (melanophages).

Histopathology

The characteristic pattern is an acanthotic epidermis with lentiginous proliferation and atypical melanocytes. Neoplastic melanocytes proliferate mainly in crista profunda intermedia. Nests of tumor cells develop, especially at the tips of the rete ridges, and they may become confluent with bridging. In the vertical growth phase the tumor often develops spindle cells.

References

118; 128; 140; 207; 238; 239; 240

Actinic Elastosis

▶ Elastosis.

Actinic Keratosis

Synonyms

Synonyms for actinic keratosis are keratosis actinica, keratosis solaris, and keratosis senilis.

Definition

Actinic keratosis consists of flat or elevated, verrucous, keratotic papules, initially 3–6 mm in size (Fig. 2), occur predominantly in chronically sun-exposed areas. They have an erythematous base and are usually covered by scales. Over time the lesions enlarge gradually and may progress into squamous cell carcinoma.

Surface Microscopy

The erythematous type has a rough, broken, and partially transparent scaly surface overlying red patches which are permeated by teleangiectases originating from the horizontally arranged subpapillary plexus (Fig. 3). Irregular linear–polymorphous blood vessels become visible and pinpoint-like short capillaries within the papillary dermis are diminished or absent. In the keratotic types the keratotic scales become thicker and the reddened patches are no longer visible. Instead, a yellowish, dirty-brown, or gray-black scaly surface may be seen. When the scale is removed, a reddened and partly fissured surface is exposed, consisting of irregularly arranged polymorphous, thrombosed, and dilated vessels, as seen in bowenoid type. The periphery of the lesions reveals a reddish rim of ectatic vessels. On occasion, the keratinization may become so prominent that a cutaneous horn develops (cornu

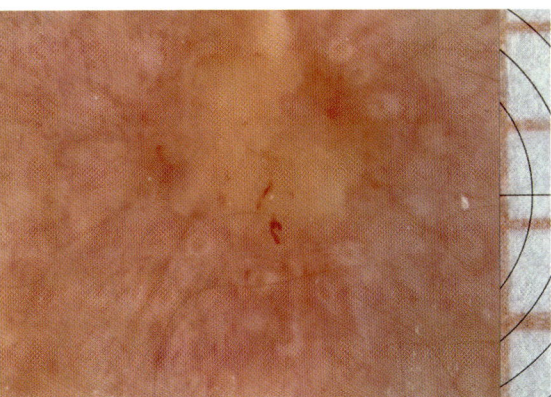

Fig. 2 Pigmented actinic keratosis on the cheek shows interfollicular gray granules (melanophages) and irregularly arranged whitish areas (fibrosis, elastosis)

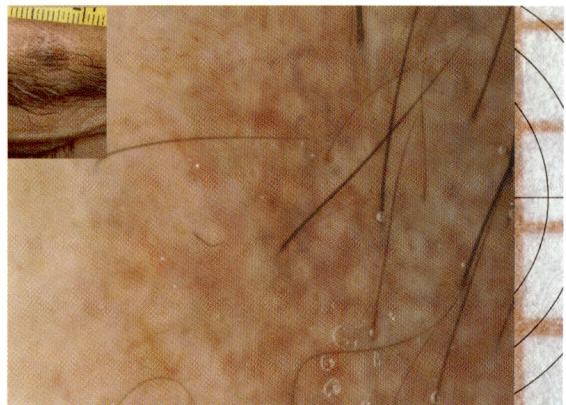

Fig. 3 Erythematous actinic keratosis on the forehead shows a yellowish hyperkeratotic plaque in the center of the lesion and irregular linear–polymorphous vessels in the surrounding area. Note the fine thrombotic vessels overlying the plaque

cutaneum type). In the lichen planus-type (lichenoid actinic keratosis; Fig. 4) the features resemble those of a lichen planus consisting of gray streaks, multiple blue-gray dots, granular dust (dermal melanophages), and diffuse hyperpigmented areas (pigment incontinence). The rarest and most variant feature is the pigmented actinic keratosis, which is characterized by a brown to slate-gray, often asymmetrically pigmented pseudonetwork pattern. The slate-gray colored melanophages are confined to the upper dermis, with aggregation in interfollicular spaces.

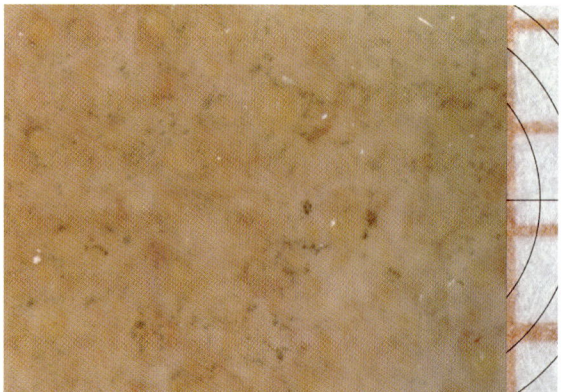

Fig. 4 Lichenoid actinic keratosis on the eyebrow with interfollicular blue-gray branched streaks, light-brown pigmented areas (pigment incontinence), and dilated vessels

Histopathology

In the hypertrophic (acanthotic), atrophic, and bowenoid variants, the abnormal epidermal proliferation results in hyperkeratotic, parakeratotic, dyskeratotic, and/or acantholytic changes. The arrangement of the atypical keratinocytes is disturbed and irregular. In the upper dermis, there is actinic elastosis, often with a chronic inflammatory infiltrate.

References

58; 72; 105; 138; 178; 198; 223; 241; 246; 281

Addison's Disease

▶ Hyperpigmentation

Adnexae

Cutaneous appendages include nails, hairs, sebaceous glands (follicular plug and opening), and both eccrine (eccrine pores) and apocrine sweat glands. The terminal hair follicles extend into the subcutis. Vellus hair follicles cover most of the body, except the palms, the plantar region, and the mucous membranes.

Age Spot

▶ Seborrheic keratoses.

Aggregated Melanocytic Nevus

▶ Agminate melanocytic nevus.

Agminate Melanocytic Nevus

Synonym

The synonym for agminate melanocytic nevus is aggregated melanocytic nevus.

Definition

Agminate melanocytic nevus is a melanocytic lesion which consists of multiple, smaller, individual lesions of a specific melanocytic type (common, blue, Spitz, or dysplastic nevi, etc.; Figs. 5, 6) grouped together, usually in a segmental or zosteriform arrangement. Some of them resemble those seen in the LEOPARD syndrome, with or without associated diseases such as cardiomyopathy, pulmonary stenosis, and ocular hypertelorism.

References

172; 298

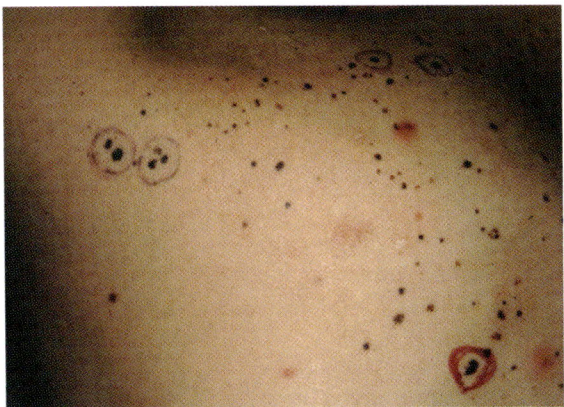

Fig. 5 Agminate (aggregated) melanocytic nevi in a segmental arrangement on the scapular region. The nevi surrounded by circular markings are dysplastic ones

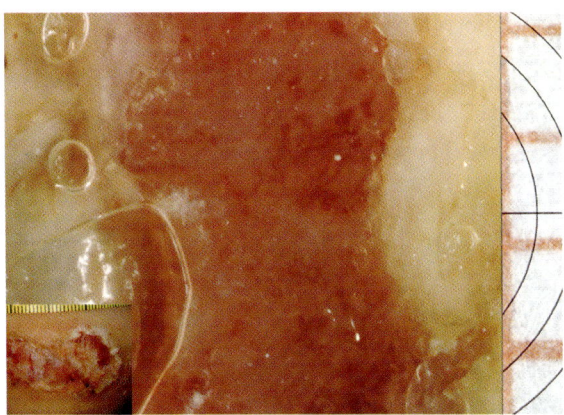

Fig. 7 Amelanotic melanoma on the sole (Clark level IV, Breslow thickness 4.2 mm) represents irregular polymorphous and glomerular vessels

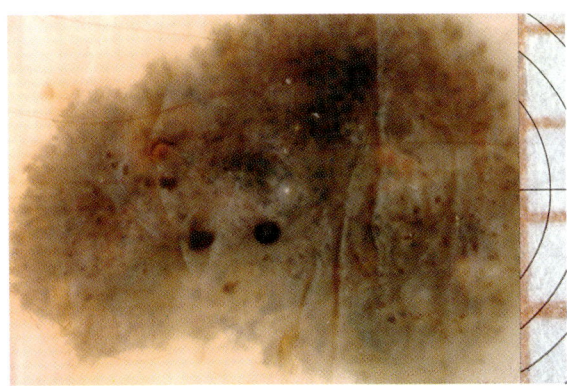

Fig. 6 Individual dysplastic compound nevus from the same patient shows a multicomponent pattern with slate-gray and brown dots, perifollicular hyperpigmentations, and light-brown globules at the border

Alabaster–Gypseous Lacunae

▶ Plaster-of-Paris-like lacunae.

Amelanotic and Hypomelanotic Melanoma

Synonym

The synonym for amelanotic and hypomelanotic melanoma is amelanotic melanoma.

Definition

Amelanotic melanoma (AMM; Fig. 7) is a flat to nodular malignant melanocytic tumor lacking grossly visible melanin (amelanotic). Some AMM may show pink plaques or light-brown pigmentation (hypomelanotype), due to either regression or the presence of defective melanocytes. Amelanotic areas may reveal pigmentation at microscopic level (partially pigmented).

Surface Microscopy

In a partially pigmented melanoma, the hypopigmented areas with pinpoint or dotted vessels are located at the periphery of the lesion, whereas in the amelanotic lesions the entire lesion shows a vascularized pattern composed of irregular polymorphous vessels, irregular hairpin-like-shaped vessels, milky-red or blue-red areas, and glomerular vessels. The absence of whitish halos (representing the layer of viable keratinocytes) surrounding blood vessels is a typical phenomenon in malignant melanomas. Often white scarlike areas and subtle remnants of melanin pigment are observed.

References

131; 160; 276; 310

Amiodaron-induced Pigmentation

▶ Hyperpigmentation.

Angiokeratoma

Definition

Angiokeratoma (Fig. 8), a benign superficial vascular ectasia within the papillary dermis, is associated with overlying hyperkeratosis. Early solitary lesion presents as verrucous carcinoma with a dark-red to purple color, 2- to 10-mm-sized papule, or as nodules.

Surface Microscopy

Some early lesions are very similar to hemangiomas, consisting of multiple, well-demarcated, red to red-blue, round to oval lacunae. The later lesions often appear with an overlying whitish-yellow hue and a translucent jelly-like periphery, resulting from the acanthotic and hyperkeratotic epidermis. The lesion may become thrombosed, appearing as a confluent blue-black pigmentation that is sharply demarcated at the periphery.

Histopathology

Angiokeratomas are not true angiomas but rather teleangiectatic vessels within the papillary dermis. The characteristic findings consist of markedly dilated, thin-walled vascular channels. The overlying epidermis is acanthotic with hyperkeratosis. Extravasation of erythrocytes and thrombosis are also common features.

References

126; 136

Angioma

▶ Hemangiomas.

Angiosarcoma

Definition

Angiosarcoma is a malignant proliferation of endothelial cells of lymphovascular origin with variable biological grade (Fig. 9).

Surface Microscopy

There are mainly milky-red to brownish-red areas without distinct borders, individual lagoons (lacunae), polymorphous vessels, and blood-filled fissures.

Histopathology

Initially, angioplastic changes are found mimicking capillary-like structures lined with atypical endothelium. Later, destructive infiltration by solid masses of highly atypical polymorphous spindle or epithelial cells, associated with erythrocyte extravasation and ulceration, occurs.

References

13; 58; 298

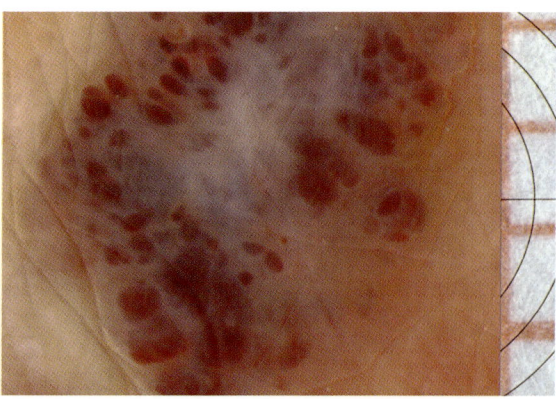

◘ **Fig. 8** Early angiokeratoma on the scapular region shows multiple red-blue oval lacunae and a whitish yellow hue in the center

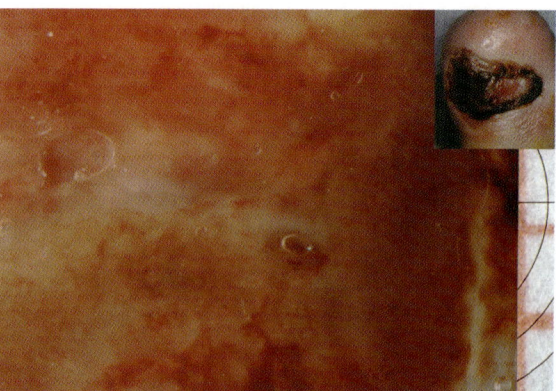

◘ **Fig. 9** Subungual angiosarcoma shows an ill-defined milky-red to brownish-red structureless area with multiple bleeding vessels and blood-filled fissures

Annular–Granular Pattern

Synonyms

Synonyms for the annular–granular pattern are Cognetta sign, rhomboidal structures, and pseudotrabeculae of melanophages.

Definition

The annular–granular pattern is a pseudonetwork (not due to pigmentation of rete ridges; the central holes exhibit pilosebaceous ostia) on adult facial skin created by openings of hyperpigmented asymmetric follicles and pigment-free sweat gland openings intersected by interfollicular slate-gray to dark-brown granules and dots.

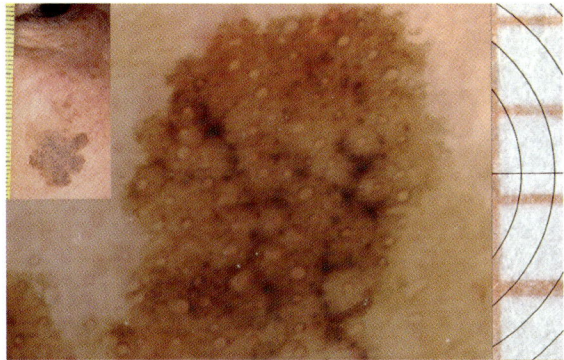

Fig. 10 Lentigo maligna in the zygomatic region shows an annular–granular pattern with dark rhomboidal structures and numerous follicular openings surrounded by a rim of hyperpigmentation (pigmented basal lamina and outer root sheath)

Occurrence

The annular–granular pattern occurs as lentigo maligna (Figs. 10, 11), lentigo maligna melanoma, senile lentigo, pigmented actinic keratosis (Fig. 12), melanocytic nevi (very rarely), melanosis, melasma.

Surface Microscopy

The annular–granular pattern shows an irregular brown macule composed of multiple blue-gray dots, slate-gray granules (melanophages), and globules which are aggregated around variably more or less hyperpigmented follicles creating inward-forming intersecting (interfollicular) streaks (pseudotrabeculae), dark rhomboidal structures, and pseudonetworks. The pilosebaceous follicles are frequently surrounded by a rim of hyperpigmentation. The asymmetric pigmented rims of the orificia correspond to an irregular extension of atypical melanocytes within individual hair follicles.

Histopathology

The rete ridges are flat to absent, and only rarely on the facial areas. The basal layer of the epidermis contains lentiginous proliferation of nevocytes, atypical melanocytes, with occasional upward migration. There is an increased deposition of melanin within keratinocytes. The upper dermis has melanin in aggregations of macrophages. In lentigo maligna and lentigo maligna melanoma there is an uneven extension and descent of atypical melanocytes into pilosebaceous skin appendages. When the basement membrane zone is invaded by the tumor cells, the lesion is designated as a lentigo maligna melanoma.

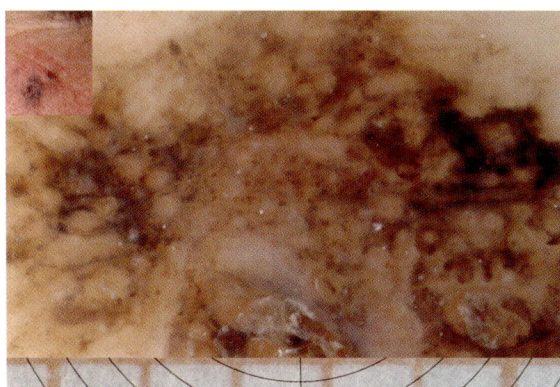

Fig. 11 Lentigo maligna melanoma (Clark level II, Breslow thickness 0.38 mm) in the zygomatic region shows an annular–granular pattern with dark rhomboidal structures, slate-gray dots, and a gray-blue veil

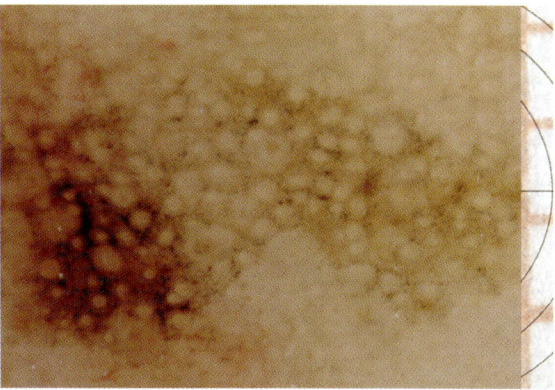

Fig. 12 Actinic keratosis (nose). An annular–granular pattern with slate-gray to dark-brown dots and short streaks around the follicle openings is seen

References

58; 188; 245; 271; 298

Apocrine Sweat Gland

Apocrine sweat glands develop in association with hair follicles and undergo enlargement and secretory development at puberty. They are primarily distributed in the axillary, genital, and mammary region producing sweat with a characteristic odor.

Arborizing Pattern

▶ Arborizing vessels.

Arborizing Telangiectasis

▶ Arborizing vessels.

Arborizing Vessels

Synonyms

Synonyms for arborizing vessels are tree-like telangiectasis, tree-like branching, arborizing telangiectasis, and arborizing pattern.

Definition

Arborizing vessels are tubular vessels with a large diameter, branching irregularly in a tree-like pattern (Fig. 13).

Occurrence

The occurrence is of basal cell carcinoma (Fig. 14), rarely seen in melanomas and benign nevi, UV-light damaged facial skin.

Surface Microscopy

Bright-red branching tree-like structures running parallel to the skin surface (vessels of the subpapillary dermal plexus, i.e., superficial dermal plexus), they are located on the surface of the lesion just below the epidermis.

References

160; 187; 217; 218

Area of Polymorphic Ectatic Vessels

Synonym

An area of polymorphic ectatic vessels is an area with unevenly arranged capillaries of various morphologies.

Definition

Areas of polymorphic ectatic vessels are round to oval or polygonal irregularly distributed vascular areas within melanocytic lesions showing polymorphic, dotted, and/or linear dilated vessels running parallel to the skin surface (Fig. 15).

Occurrence

Areas of polymorphic ectatic vessels are common in primary malignant melanomas, indicating an area of

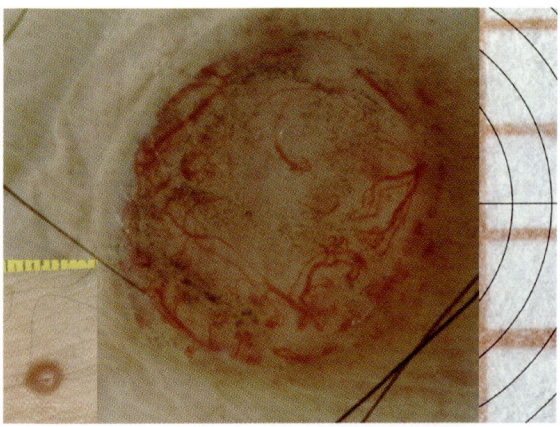

■ **Fig. 13** Arborizing vessels of various calibers are present within a basal cell carcinoma (same patient as in Fig. 1, higher magnification)

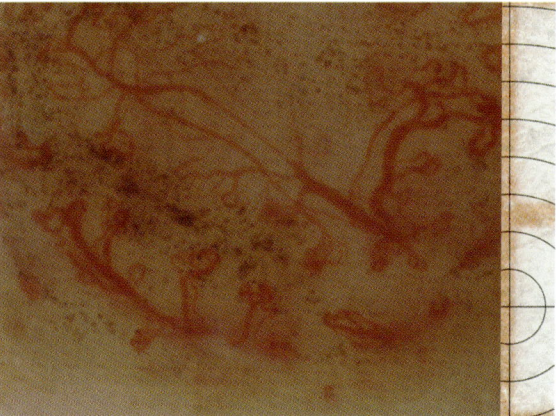

■ **Fig. 14** Pigmented basal cell carcinoma (popliteal region). The absence of a pigmented network with arborizing vessels and brown pigment granules without associated pigment networks define this lesion

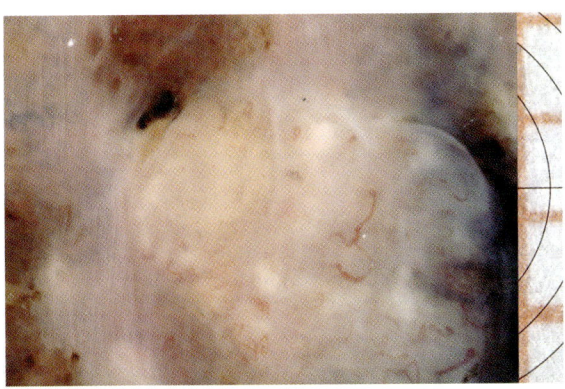

Fig. 15 Superficial spreading melanoma on the sternal region (Clark level III, Breslow thickness 1.2 mm) presenting with a hypopigmented area with polymorphic and aneurysmatic vessels

the vertical growth phase (with a specificity of 89% and a sensitivity of 41% when referring to melanocytic lesions), and in cutaneous melanoma metastases.

Surface Microscopy

The vessels display a broad range of variation in size and diameter within the hypopigmented areas including dilated, aneurysmal, and polymorphic changes (resembling Greek minuscules). In some of the pigment cell tumors the neovascularization can occur as a circumscribed amelanotic area of dotted and regularly arranged loops without any background structure (so-called naked papillae).

References

11; 16; 231; 252; 257; 260; 261; 262; 263; 300

Area of Target Globules

▶ Target globules.

Area with Central Papillary Globules

▶ Target globules.

Area with Evenly Arranged Capillaries

▶ Area of polymorphic ectatic vessels.

Asymmetrical Pigmented Follicular Openings

▶ Perifollicular pigment changes.

Atrophy of the Epidermis

The normal thickness of the stratum spinosum decreases (to a few layers of cells) with concurrent diminishing of the stratum granulosum and stratum corneum, and is associated with flattened epidermal rete ridges. Under surface microscopy the atrophic epidermis becomes more translucent.

Atypical Nevus

▶ Dysplastic nevus.

Atypical Pigment Network

Synonym
The synonym for atypical pigment network is prominent/irregular pigmented network.

Definition
An atypical pigment network is a black, brown, or gray network of variably thick lines with irregular holes.

Occurrence
Atypical pigment network occurs as malignant melanomas, dysplastic/atypical nevi (Figs. 16, 17), and, only rarely, benign nevi.

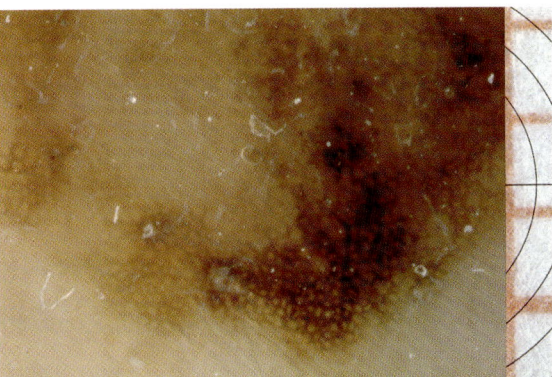

Fig. 16 Dysplastic nevus on the neck, characterized by brown to black irregular network of fragmented unevenly thickened and compact trabeculae

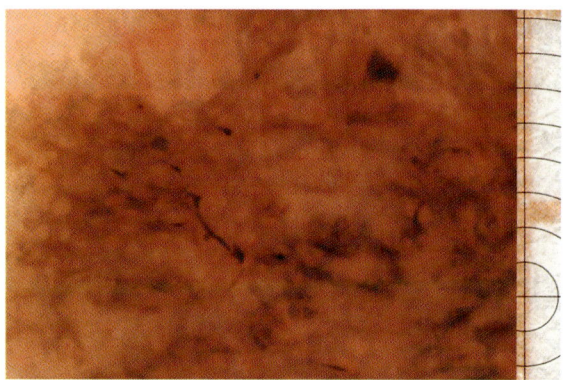

Fig. 17 Dysplastic nevus on the scapular region displaying broadened and hyperpigmented streaks and black dots

Surface Microscopy

Atypical pigment network is characterized by a prominent, irregular mesh-like network of variable sized, broadened, and hyperpigmented lines (grids), with often an abrupt cut-off at the periphery.

References

26; 82; 188

Atypical Vascular Pattern

Definition

Atypical vascular pattern consists of vascular structures which are irregularly distributed throughout a lesion with linear–irregular, polymorphous, or dotted vessels perpendicular to the skin surface (Fig. 18) and are not clearly associated with regression structures.

Occurrence

Atypical vascular pattern occurs as hypopigmented or amelanotic melanomas, malignant melanomas (vertical growth phase), and cutaneous malignant melanoma metastases.

References

26; 170

Auspitz Sign

Synonyms

Synonyms for Auspitz sign (Fig. 19) are Auspitz's phenomenon and focal bleeding phenomenon.

Definition

By removing the superficial skin layer of a psoriatic lesion, the capillaries in the dermal papillae are damaged, resulting in punctate bleeding.

Surface Microscopy

After removal of the scaly material and the superficial layer of the epidermis, the lesion demonstrates multiple homogeneous convoluted coiled papillary angiectasis (ectatic capillary loops in the stratum papillare) and with punctate hemorrhage.

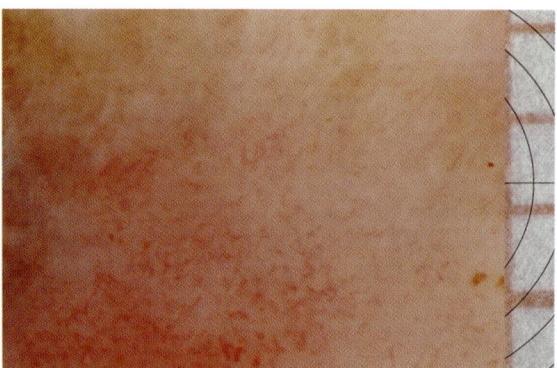

Fig. 18 Superficial spreading melanoma (Clark level IV, Breslow thickness 1.8 mm). The area with an atypical vascular pattern is characterized by a combination of linear–irregular and dotted vessels

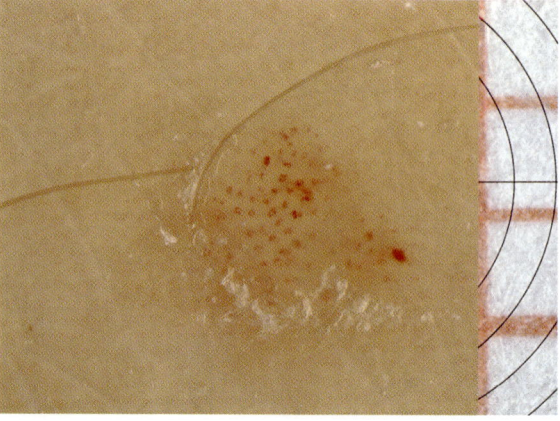

Fig. 19 Primary lesion in psoriasis vulgaris exanthematicus after scraping off the surface scale shows ectatic capillary loops and punctate hemorrhage

References
58; 104; 308; 311

Autoimmunogenic Keratinocytolysis

Definition

Autoimmune diseases or immunological reactions of the skin, e.g., lupus erythematosus (Fig. 20), chronicus discoides, tumor-induced immune reactions, are associated with abnormal keratinization. Using surface microscopy, the small, circular, whitish rims noted within the outer root sheath of the pilosebaceous apparatus indicate an abnormal keratinolytic process. This dermoscopic phenomenon may help to detect the initial stages of an autoimmunogenic disorder.

Reference

262

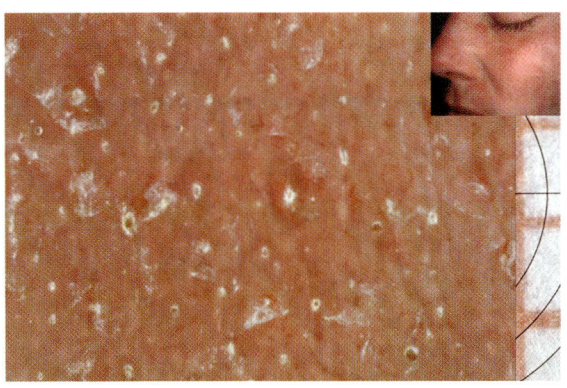

Fig. 20 Initial stage of facial discoid lupus erythematosus represents multiple whitish rims of the follicular openings

AVP

▶ Atypical vascular pattern

Balloon Cell Nevus

Definition

A balloon cell nevus is an intradermal or compound melanocytic lesion that consists of enlarged epithelial melanocytes with an expanded, clear, often vacuolated cytoplasm (balloon cells), and with a uniform, centrally positioned nucleus.

Surface Microscopy

There are branched streaks, dots, structureless areas, multiple light-colored holes, and pseudohorncysts within a brown pigmented macule.

Histopathology

The ballooned nevus cells are often distributed in asymmetrical fashion. They are situated mostly in nests in the dermis or at the dermoepidermal junction without apparent mitotic figures.

References

5; 118; 298

Basal Cell Carcinoma

Synonyms

Synonyms for basal cell carcinoma are basal cell epithelioma and basal cell cancer.

Definition

Basal cell carcinoma is a malignant, characteristically non-metastasizing epithelial tumor originating from the basal cells in the epidermis and the hair follicles (Figs. 21, 22). It presents a local exophytic growth, endophytic infiltration, or both, with different clinical manifestations (superficial, solid–nodular, pigmented, ulcerating, morpheiform, keloidal, cystic) indicating varying histological growth patterns.

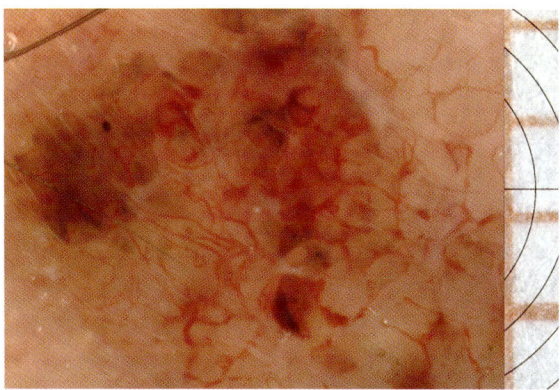

Fig. 21 Preauricular pigmented adenoid basal cell carcinoma demonstrates arborizing telangiectasia, leaf-like areas, and a blue-gray globule

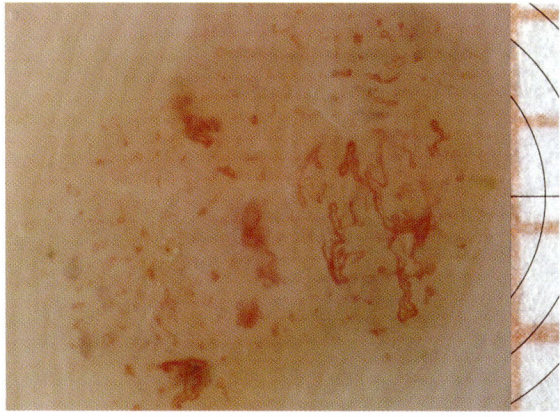

Fig. 22 Superficial non-pigmented basal cell carcinoma on the back shows glomerular, arborizing, and dotted vessels on a reddish-yellowish background

Surface Microscopy

The findings are characterized by the presence of irregular central hypopigmentation, irregular blotches, and arborizing blood vessels (tree-like branching) of different diameters, without an obvious pigment network. The arborizing vessels with numerous branches are situated along the surface of the tumor. The criteria for the pigmented type include the following features: leaf-like areas of gray-brown to slate-gray color; gray-black and blue-gray ovoid nests; multiple blue-gray globules and spoke-wheel-like areas. Some of the lesions may contain pseudohorn cysts.

Histopathology

Basal cell carcinomas are characterized by dermal proliferation of atypical cells that resemble epidermal basal cells showing a palisade-like arrangement at the periphery of the tumor mass. Characteristic peritumoral stromal clefting is present. Melanin pigment may be present either in the tumor lobules, in the tumor stroma, or both.

References

38; 58; 66; 82; 187; 318

Basal Cell Papilloma

▶ Seborrheic keratoses.

Basal Layer

▶ Stratum basale.

Basic Pattern of Polymorphic and/or Aneurysmatic Vessels

▶ Polymorphic angiectatic base pattern.

Basic Structures

There are mainly six surface microscopic basic structures that can be identified without difficulty: the shape of the horny layer; the rete ridges of the stratum Malpighii; the dermal papillae corresponding with the "holes" of the network pattern; blood vessels of the skin (central capillary loops in the dermal papillae, superficial, and deep vascular plexus running parallel to the skin surface, vertical connecting vessels); the pilosebaceous apparatus (follicular openings); and the eccrine and apocrine sweat glands openings.

Bathing Trunk Nevus

▶ Congenital melanocytic nevus.

Becker's Nevus

▶ Melanosis neviformis.

Benign Juvenile Melanoma

▶ Spitz nevus.

Benign Lichenoid Keratosis

▶ Seborrheic keratoses.

Black Dots

▶ Dots.

Black Heel

Definition

Black heel (Fig. 23) is a variable-sized cutaneous hemorrhage of the heel caused by trauma from sporting activities or poorly fitting sport shoes.

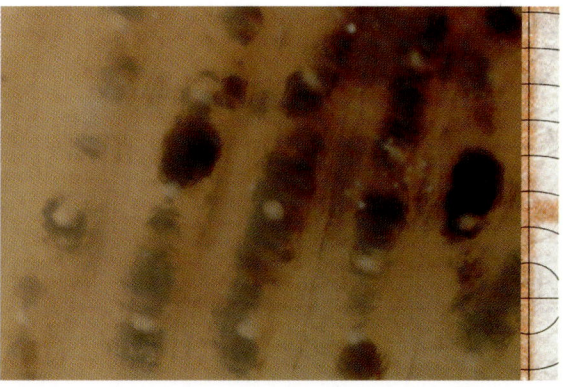

◻ Fig. 23 Black heel mimicks the parallel ridge pattern

Surface Microscopy

Black heel consists of multiple yellow-red to reddish-black linear or round to oval areas (due to bleeding) with smooth margins arranged mainly on the ridges, slightly mimicking the parallel ridge pattern (in red). The hypopigmented openings of the sweat ducts are found within the darker zones. There are tiny red satellites at the periphery.

Reference

240

Blood Lakes

► Ovoid blood lakes.

Blood Sinuses

► Lacunae.

Blood Spots, Nail Unit

Synonym

The synonym for blood spots is subungual hemorrhage.

Definition

A blood spot is a subungual hemorrhage that represents sharply demarcated blood spots and satellite blood spots that are characterized by a homogeneous coloration (absence of brown lines; Fig. 24). Recent lesions are purple and round. They become brown and have a more linear pattern in long-standing lesions. If the blood is heavily clotted, the spots become red-black in color.

Reference

302

Blotches

Synonyms

Synonyms for blotches are black lamella and irregular blotches.

Definition

There are large concentrations of melanin pigment localized throughout the epidermis and/or dermis, visually obscuring the underlying structures.

Occurrence

The occurrence is of lentigines (Fig. 25), benign nevi, and malignant melanomas (irregular and asymmetrically distributed within the lesion).

Surface Microscopy

The surface microscopy consists of regular or irregular structureless areas of localized or diffuse pigmentation of black, brown, and/or gray color obscuring the underlying structures.

References

26; 82; 142; 180; 279; 323

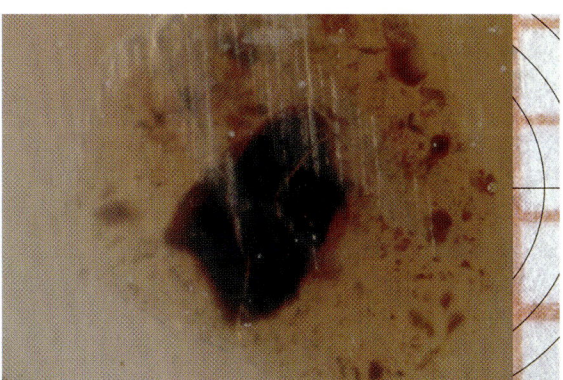

◘ **Fig. 24** Subungual hemorrhage on an adult's first toenail (long-standing lesion) represents well-demarcated round, ovoid, or polycyclic reddish-brown to dark-brown blood spots

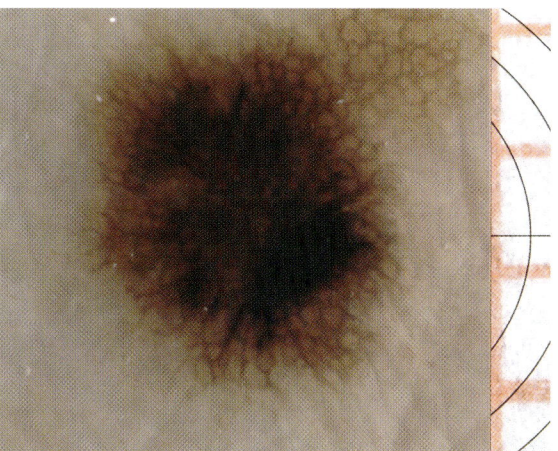

◘ **Fig. 25** Lentigo simplex in the umbilical region characterized by black blotches in the center and a regular network at the periphery

Blue Nevus

Synonym

The synonym for blue nevis is nevus ceruleus.

Definition

Blue nevi are flat or slightly elevated blue (steel blue, dark blue, blue-black, blue-gray), smooth-surfaced macules or papules or smooth-surfaced macules which are formed by dendritic or epithelioid melanocytes in the mid- to lower dermis (Fig. 26). Proliferation of melanocytes that does not usually eventuate in nests is usually confined to the dermis only.

Surface Microscopy

There is a homogeneous pattern throughout the entire lesion with a diffuse steel-blue to blue-gray pigmentation fading into the surrounding skin in absence of a network or branched streaks. Some blue nevi may develop epidermal hyperpigmentation (e.g., a brown veil) and some have a whitish scar-like appearance. Individual blue globules and dots are also observed. Fibrosing blue nevi may contain focal areas of confluent hypopigmentation due to increased collagen deposition within reticular dermis.

Histopathology

There is a loss of rete ridges. Nodular proliferation of spindle-shaped, fibroblast-like or dendritic melanocytes are distributed between the collagen fibers in the dermis. The melanocytes are entirely intradermal, and they do not progress from junctional to compound stages. Melanophages are numerous, associated with variable fibrosis.

References

82; 118; 139; 206; 223; 232

Blue-gray Area

▶ Blue-white veil.

Blue-gray Globules in Absence of a Pigment Network

Synonym

The synonym for blue-gray area is multiple blue-gray globules.

Definition

Blue-gray globules are characterized by blue-gray round, spherical, and well-circumscribed structures (> 0.1 mm in diameter; Fig. 27), in absence of a pigment network.

Occurrence

Basal cell carcinoma is the occurrence (with a specificity of 97% for pigmented basal cell carcinoma), in a rare variant of pigmented seborrheic keratoses.

Surface Microscopy

The surface microscopy consists of multiple blue-gray spherical shapes usually not connected to a pigmented tumor body.

Histopathology

There are scattered focal collections of melanin pigment within the tumor nests.

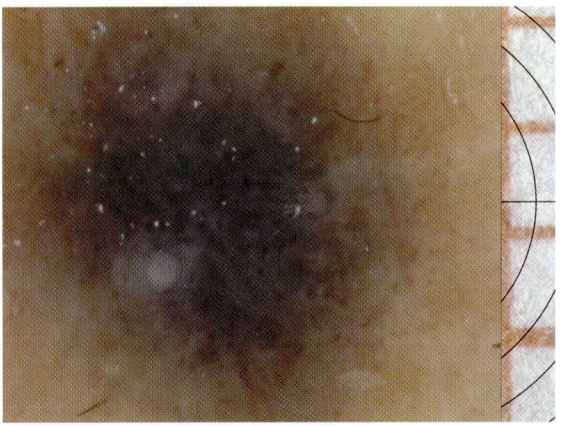

Fig. 26 A blue nevus shows homogeneous slate-gray to blue pigmentation

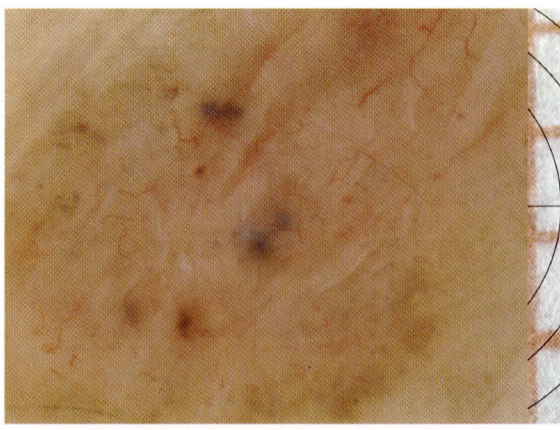

Fig. 27 Multiple blue-gray globules in a pigmented basal cell carcinoma of the trunk

References

142; 187; 188; 280; 298

Blue-gray Granules

▶ Multiple blue-gray dots.

Blue-gray or Slate-gray Reticular Pattern

Synonym

The synonym for blue-gray or slate-gray reticular pattern is slate-gray remnants of a network.

Definition

The blue-gray or slate-gray color of network fragments or remnants refers to aggregates of poorly or non-pigmented atypical melanocytes overlying broadened and elongated pigmented rete ridges at the border or within a malignant melanocytic lesion (Fig. 28).

Occurrence

They occur as malignant melanomas.

Reference

257

Blue-gray Reticular Pattern

▶ Blue-gray or slate-gray reticular pattern.

Blue-in-Pink Area

Synonym

Blue-in-pink area is a synonym for blue-red area.

Definition

These entities are asymmetrically distributed oval to polygonal or poorly defined blue-and pink-tinged structures of 0.2–0.4 mm, rarely > 1.0 mm in diameter located within the melanocytic lesions (Figs. 29, 30).

Occurrence

They occur as malignant melanomas (with a specificity of > 80% and a sensitivity of 36%), dysplastic/atypical nevi, combined nevi, and Spitz nevi.

Surface Microscopy

A blue-in-pink zone is seen as blue to blue-gray streaks, dots or aggregated granules on a pinkish background. It is localized at the periphery or irregularly near the center.

Histopathology

The histopathology shows blue to blue-gray dots and streaks tending to vary in size and shape are due to proliferating melanocytic nests situated at the dermo-epidermal junction, or in the papillary dermis. Blue or blue-gray granules may include free melanin, fine melanin particles or melanin in macrophages, or free melanin in the deep papillary or reticular dermis. The pinkish background is due to variable neovascularization within an area of fibrosis and regression.

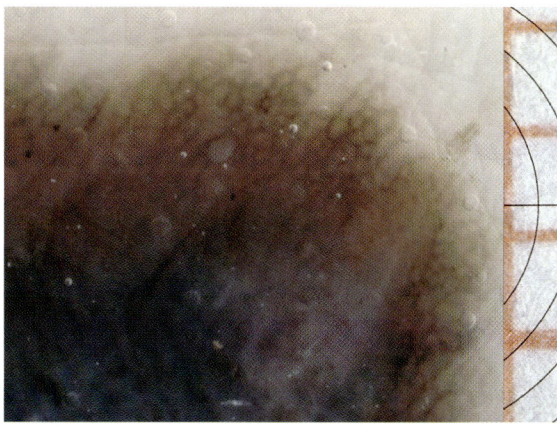

■ **Fig. 28** Nodular melanoma on the trunk (Clark level IV, Breslow thickness 3.5 mm) shows a slate-gray reticular pattern at the border of the lesion

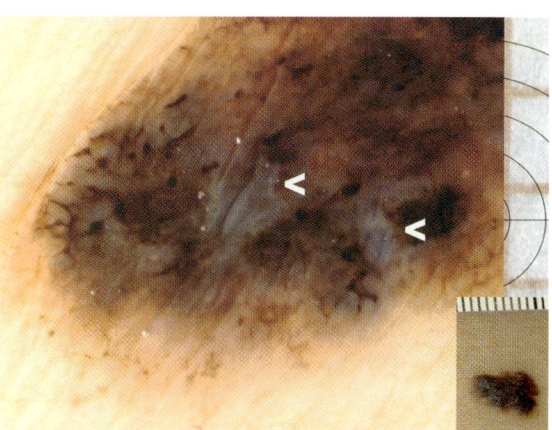

■ **Fig. 29** Superficial spreading melanoma (Clark level III, Breslow thickness 0.66 mm). Peripheral blue-in-pink areas are present at or near the edge of the lesion (*arrowheads*)

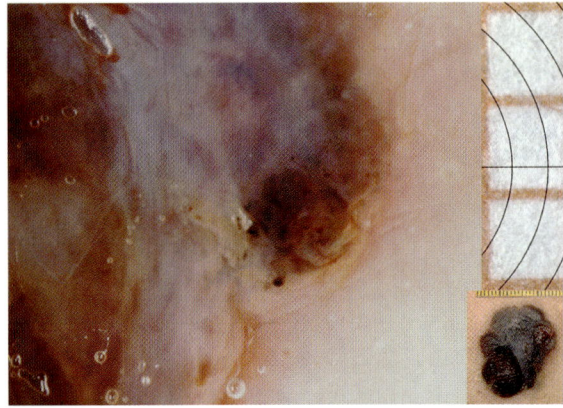

Fig. 30 Unclassified malignant melanoma (Clark level IV, Breslow thickness 7.6 mm). Peripheral blue-in-pink area is located at the edge of the lesion

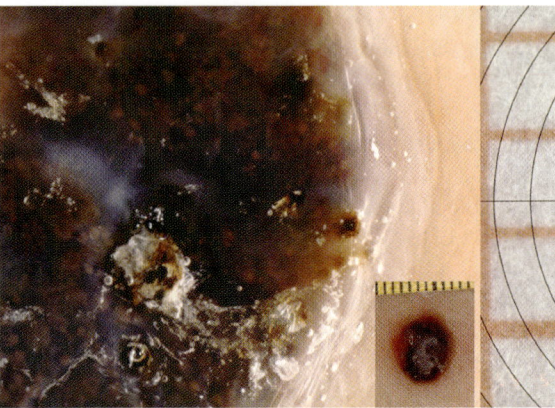

Fig. 31 Nodular malignant melanoma (Clark level IV, Breslow thickness 2.2 mm) exhibits blue-white veil in the center

References

142; 143; 231; 257; 260; 262; 278; 298

Blue-white Veil

Synonyms

Synonyms for blue-white veil are gray-blue area/veil, blue-whitish area, bluish opaque veil, whitish veil, and milky way.

Definition

Blue-white veil is an irregular indistinct configuration of a blue pigmentation with an overlying opaque or white "ground-glass hue," not associated with red-blue lacunes (hemangiomas).

Occurrence

Blue-white veil occurs as malignant melanomas (specificity >95%, sensitivity >30%, in invasive melanomas >50%; Fig. 31), blue nevi (homogeneous steel-blue color filling out the whole lesion; Fig. 32), melanoma metastases, Spitz nevi (Fig. 33), and recurrent melanocytic nevi.

Surface Microscopy

Non-uniform, diffuse, structureless, confluent bluish-whitish hue (white "ground glass" appearance) sometimes with underlying scar-like areas (regression pattern) and/or collections of scattered melanophages (peppered appearance). In contrast to most blue nevi, the whitish veil or film due to a compact orthokeratosis cannot occupy the entire lesion due to a compact orthokeratosis.

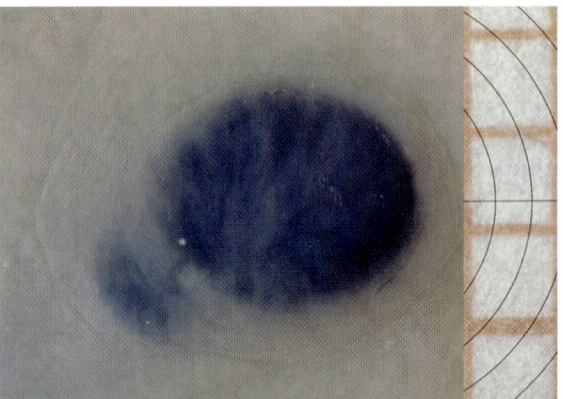

Fig. 32 Cutaneous malignant melanoma in-transit metastasis in the scapular region shows a homogeneous blue-white veil mimicking blue nevus. There is an absence of network, branched streaks, and globules

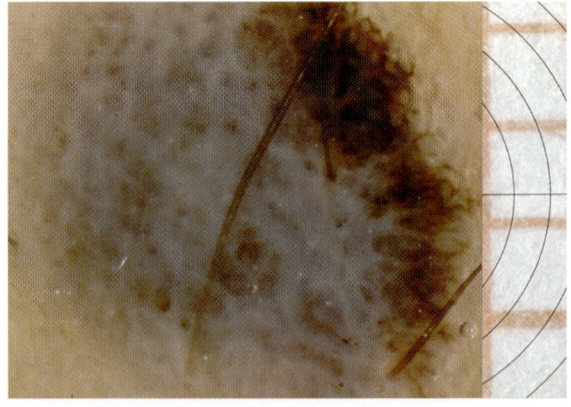

Fig. 33 Spitz nevus. Blue-white veil in the center of the lesion. In addition, there are underlying blue-gray to gray-brown sacculi (globules) and a pigment network (*right* side of the lesion)

Histopathology

Aggregates of heavily pigmented atypical melanocytes and/or melanophages as well as free melanin (blue color) are located in the papillary dermis associated with an acanthotic and thickened orthokeratotic epidermis and focal hypergranulosis.

References

21; 31; 56; 154; 179; 186; 188; 278; 280; 298; 323

Border

Synonyms

Synonyms for border are edge and lesion edge.

Definition

Border is the edge or the shape of the border of a pigmented lesion (Figs. 34, 35). The edge may provide important diagnostic information.

Surface Microscopy

In most cases of benign nevi the network thins out towards the periphery and enters into the normal skin. If an abrupt cut-off of the network involves the total circumference of a melanocytic lesion, then it may be a feature of melanoma. There are non-specific features of melanocytic malignancy such as an irregular edge and a sharp, abrupt cut-off (abrupt edge) as well as specific features such as pseudopods, radial streaming, dots/globules, and depigmentation.

References

46; 188; 270

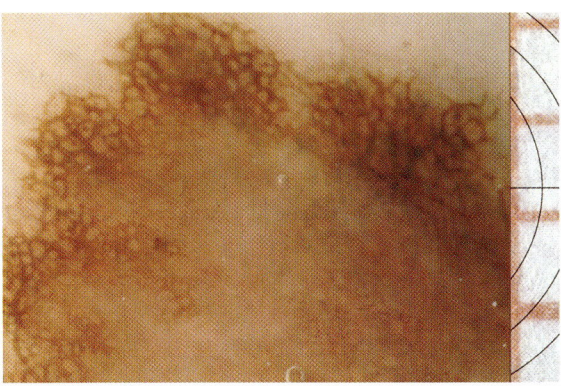

Fig. 35 A malignant melanoma in situ shows an abrupt cut-off of the pigment network

Bowen's Disease

Synonyms

Synonyms for Bowen's disease are squamous cell carcinoma in situ and dyskeratosis maligna.

Definition

Bowen's disease is an intraepidermal carcinoma with or without chronic inflammatory changes of the skin (erythematous, eczematous, psoriasiform; Fig. 36), and which has the capacity of transforming into an invasive squamous cell carcinoma.

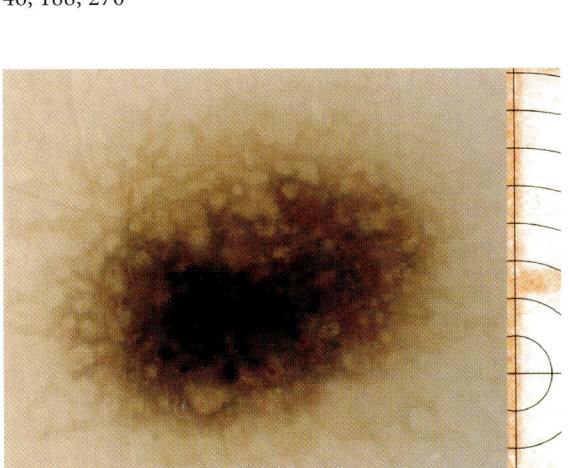

Fig. 34 A junctional nevus with an regular pigment network that gradually thins out towards the periphery

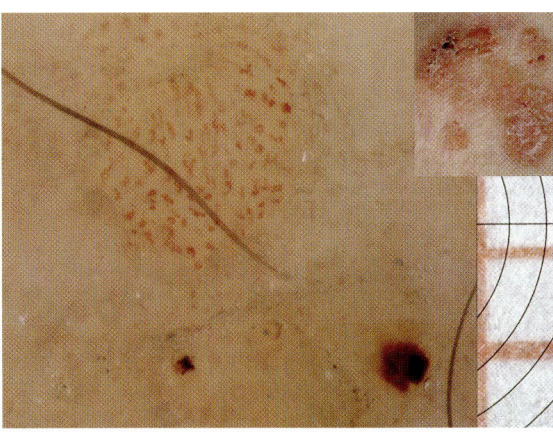

Fig. 36 Bowen's disease on the forearm represents an area of polymorphous vessels and keratin plugs with hemorrhagic crusts (*inset*)

Surface Microscopy

In Bowen's disease the dyskeratotic epidermis has lost its normal regular pattern of the rete ridges and the follicular openings. In most cases the basic pattern consists of more or less regularly distributed polymorphous (resembling Greek minuscules) and punctiform or comma-shaped capillary loops (nacked papillae) on a background tinged reddish to brownish. Many convoluted, aneurysmatic, and/or thrombosed dilated blood vessels are not visibly associated with the dermal papillae, and they go across the anatomically defined interdigitating structures. There may be a complete destruction of the pilosebaceous units and rhexis bleeding. Irregularly distributed plaques of keratin (dyskeratosis) may obscure the underlying vessels. Atrophic and regressive zones occur as structureless whitish areas. In some pigmented lesions branched streaks are seen.

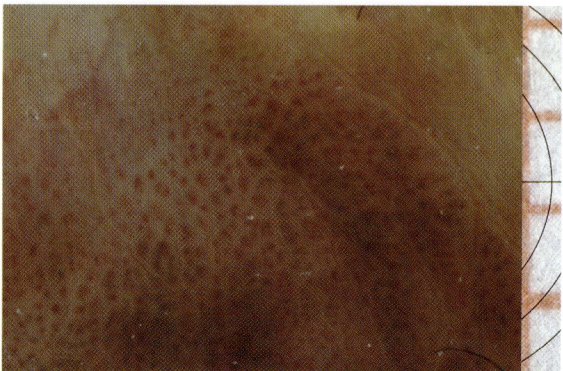

□ **Fig. 37** Bowenoid penile papule (on the corona glandis) manifests as regularly distributed ectatic vessels of the dermal papillae, some of which are surrounded by slate-gray pigmentations (melanophages)

Histopathology

In Bowen's disease the acanthotic and hyperparakeratotic epidermis has lost its normal regular pattern and is characterized by proliferation of atypical epithelial cells occupying the full thickness of the epidermis. There is also a characteristic dyskeratosis with individual cell keratinization and a pronounced stromal reaction in the upper dermis. The atypical epithelial cells have not yet invaded the basement membrane zone.

References

58; 262

Bowenoid Genital Papulosis

Synonyms

Synonyms of Bowenoid genital papulosis are pigmented penile papules and bowenoid genital papules.

Surface Microscopy

Vulval or penile papules are light-brown to slate-gray tinged (Fig. 37). The slate-gray coloration is due to melanin in the epidermis and/or abundant melanophages surrounding the capillaries of the dermal papillae. The basic pattern consists of regularly distributed polymorphous and comma-shaped capillary loops. Most capillaries are visibly associated with the dermal papillae, in contrast to Bowen's disease where the small vessels often pass over the papillary border. Aneurysmatic, convoluted, and thrombosed blood vessels have a further distinction in that they are rarely seen in bowenoid papules.

Histopathology

In the acanthotic thickened epidermis there is a proliferation of atypical cells (nuclear pleiomorphism) with viral-like cytopathological changes. Irregular thickened rete ridges are intercalated with narrow and elongated connective-tissue papillae. The overall changes resemble those of Bowen's disease-like changes, often with abundant melanin in the epithelium in the dermal papillae. A lichen planus-like inflammation can be present in the papillary dermis.

References

13; 135; 262; 312

Bowen's Carcinoma

▶ Bowen's disease.

Brain-like Appearance

▶ Fissures and ridges.

Branched Streaks

Definition

Branched streaks signify a disrupted pigment network characterized by irregularly branched streaks due to changes within a pigmented lesion.

Occurrence

Branched streaks occur as malignant melanoma, dysplastic nevus, and pigmented actinic keratosis.

Surface Microscopy

The network becomes broken up and brown to slate-gray ramifying streaks at the periphery of the lesion or in the center can be seen (Fig. 38). The color depends on the depth and width of the bridging melanocytes.

Histopathology

The histopathology shows remnants of pigmented rete ridges and bridging nests of melanocytic cells within the epidermis and papillary demis.

References

138; 142; 201; 280; 298

Broadened Network

Synonym

The synonym for broadened network is atypical broadened network.

Definition

Broadened network is an increase in the width of the "grids" or "cords" of the pigmented network found in melanocytic lesions.

Occurrence

Broadened network occurs as malignant melanomas (specificity of 86% and sensitivity of 86% for invasive melanoma), Lentigo maligna (rhomboidal structures), and very rarely benign nevi.

Surface Microscopy

The broadening of the network is usually focally found in melanoma, rather than uniformly throughout the lesion (Fig. 39). It can often be found focally at or near the edge of the lesion. Follicular openings of the face can create a pseudobroadened network in both melanocytic and non-melanocytic lesions.

Histopathology

The histopathology is expansion of melanocytic nests found at the dermo-epidermal junction.

Reference

189

Brown Background, Nail Unit

Definition

Brown background is defined as subungual pigmented lesions with a homogeneous brown coloration of the background, usually associated with overlying brown lines.

Occurrence

Brown background occurs as melanocytic nevus of the nail matrix (regular coloration and pattern with uniform parallel lines; Fig. 40), nail-unit melanoma (irregular spacing and color, disruption of parallelism, bizarre pattern with dots and globules), and subungual yellowish-brown well-demarcated psoriatic oil spots (ovoid or round in shape).

Reference

302

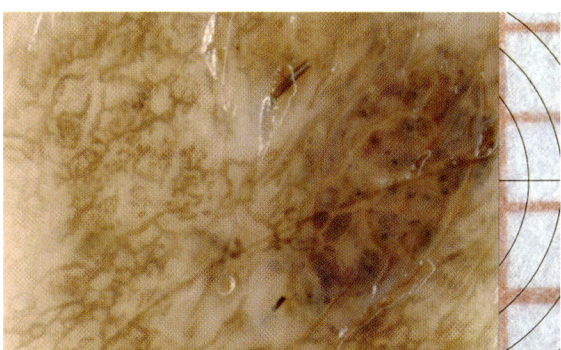

□ **Fig. 38** Congenital melanocytic nevus shows multiple branched streaks

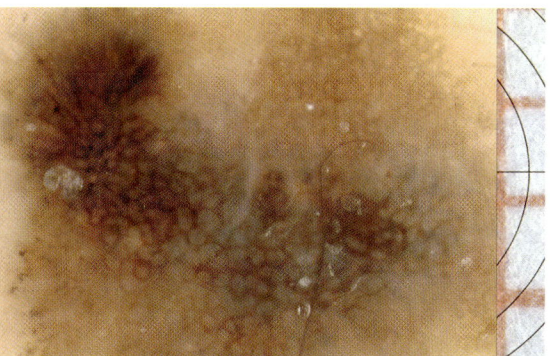

□ **Fig. 39** Superficial spreading melanoma (Clark level II, Breslow thickness 0.33 mm). This asymmetrically patterned multicolored lesion has the distinct feature of a focal broadened network and radial streaming

Brown Dots

▶ Dots.

Brown Globules

▶ Globules.

Brown/Black Dots on a Blue/Gray Background

▶ Dots.

■ **Fig. 40** Melanocytic nevus of the nail matrix shows a subungual homogeneous brown coloration of the background with overlying brown lines in a 19-year-old woman

Capillary Dot Pattern

Definition

Within skin lesions a cluster of dilated capillaries appear as an area of red dots corresponding to the central capillary loops of each dermal papilla.

References

143; 262

Capillary Reticular Pattern

Definition

Within skin lesions linear capillaries form a meshwork corresponding to the subepidermal horizontal plexus running parallel to the skin surface.

Reference

143

Capillary Sequestration

▶ Nailfold capillaries, alterations.

Central Hyperpigmented Pattern

Definition

A central hyperpigmented pattern is a basic surface microscopy pattern of melanocytic lesions with a symmetrically and strongly pigmented center that suggests a benign lesion (Fig. 41). There may be other typical criteria for melanocytic changes, e.g., peripheral network, dots, and globules present.

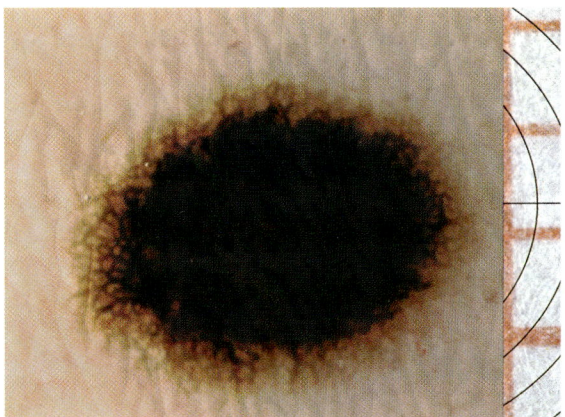

◼ **Fig. 41** Junctional nevus with a central hyperpigmented basic pattern and a regular peripheral network

Central Hypopigmented Pattern

Definition

Central hypopigmented pattern is a common pattern that consists of a symmetrically localized and mainly structureless hypopigmented regular area in the center of a melanocytic lesion that suggests a benign lesion (Fig. 42). In most cases a regular peripheral network may be present.

Cerebriform Appearance

▶ Fissures and ridges.

Cherry Hemangioma

▶ Hemangiomas.

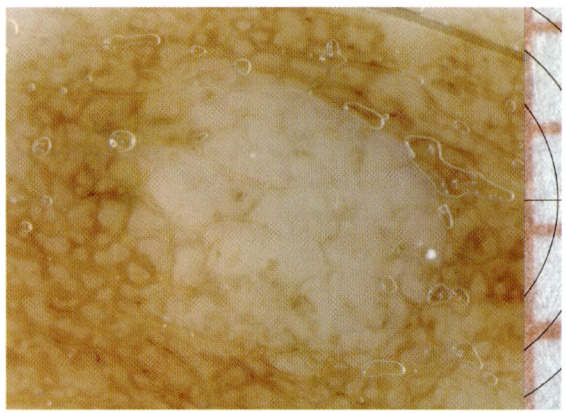

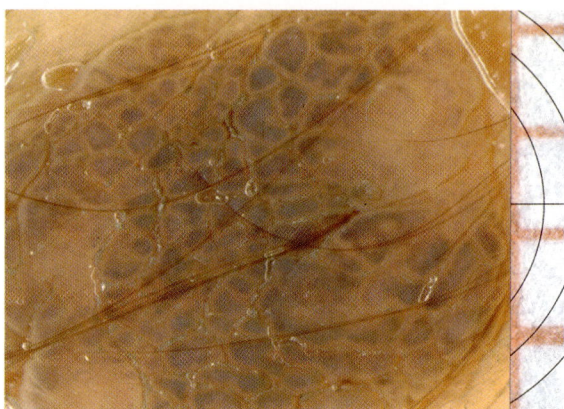

Fig. 42 Junctional nevus on the thigh represents a hypopigmented central area and a peripheral network pattern

Fig. 43 A dermal nevus shows a typical slate-gray cobblestone pattern

Clark's Nevus

▶ Dysplastic nevus.

Chloasma

▶ Hyperpigmentation.

CMN

▶ Congenital melanocytic nevus.

Cobblestone Pattern

Synonym
The synonym for cobblestone pattern is cobblestone-like pattern.

Definition
Cobblestone pattern is a composition of closely aggregated, evenly pigmented, and distributed angulated cobblestone-like "clods" or globules.

Occurrence
The occurrence is congenital melanocytic nevus, dermal nevus, and papillomatous nevus.

Surface Microscopy
In benign melanocytic lesions there are evenly distributed polygonal clods with brown, slate-gray, or black homogeneous or granular pigmentation (Fig. 43).

Histopathology
The histopathology shows heavily pigmented nests of melanocytes in the lower epidermis and the papillary dermis (intermingled with melanophages).

References
82; 298

Cockade Architecture

▶ Zonal architecture.

Cognetta Sign

▶ Annular–granular pattern.

Collision Tumors

Definition
Collision tumors signify a collision between two or more unrelated lesions, e.g., melanocytic nevi and seborrheic keratoses, infundibular cysts, or hemangiomas.

Reference
298

Color Changes

Definition

Color changes of the skin may consist of endogenous products, e.g., melanin, hemoglobin, hemosiderin, yellowish-brown bile pigments, yellow-red carotene, or yellow to brown colored lipids (lipochrome, lipofuscin). Normal epidermis appears yellowish to light red, whereas acanthotic epidermis ranges from opaque whitish-yellow to yellow-brownish or gray-brownish. Melanin can be seen in melanocytes, keratinocytes, melanophages or in various tumor cells. In melanocytic skin lesions mainly six colors can be identified: white; red; light brown; dark brown; blue-gray; and black. In the upper layers (granular layer and stratum corneum) of the epidermis melanin pigment appears black; light- to dark-brown color (depending on the concentration of melanin) is due to melanin at the dermoepidermal junction, blue to blue-gray from melanin in the papillary dermis, and melanin within the stratum reticulare looks steel blue. White color (lighter than the adjacent normal skin) is due to regressive changes (fibrosis). Red color is caused by diffuse erythema, telangiectasis, inflammation (dilated vessels), or a tumor's increased overall vascular supply (neovascularization).

References

270; 298

Combined Nevus

Definition

Combined nevus is a co-existence of two different types of melanocytic lesions, most commonly implied for the close association of a blue nevus with a common melanocytic nevus.

Surface Microscopy

Surface microscopy consists of a multicomponent pattern showing a typical pigment network of the melanocytic nevus component juxtaposed with an area of homogeneous blue-gray pigmentation, reflecting the blue nevus component (Fig. 44).

Histopathology

The dermis contains numerous dendritic, spindle-shaped, or neuroid structured (cellular blue nevus) melanocytes and melanophages in a fibrotic area. In addition, there are also nests of typical nevus cells.

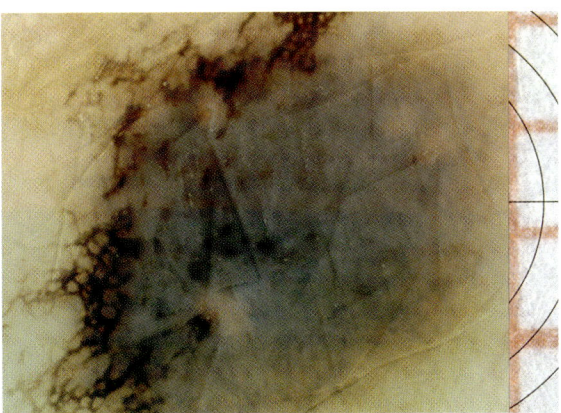

◘ **Fig. 44** Combined nevus on the scapular region shows a typical pigment network at the border partially overlying the blue-gray component

References

76; 139

Comedo-like Openings

Synonyms

The synonyms for comedo-like openings are pseudofollicular openings, crypts, blackhead-like plugs, and comedo-like plugs.

Definition

Comedo-like openings are pigmented skin lesions with non-uniform, ovoid craters that have brown or black comedo-like plugs.

Occurrence

Comedo-like openings occur as seborrheic keratosis, papillomatous melanocytic nevus, congenital melanocytic nevus, and fibroepithelial tumor (Pinkus tumor), and are occasionally seen in melanoma.

Surface Microscopy

Comedo-like openings are irregularly shaped light-brown to dark-brown round and well-demarcated concave craters filled with keratin corresponding to a morphological variant of fissures (Figs. 45, 46).

Histopathology

Histopathology shows keratin-filled invaginations of the epidermis (hyperkeratinized clefts, or pseudohorncysts).

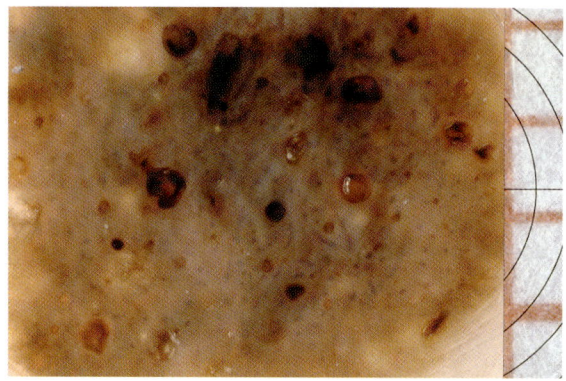

Fig. 45 A pigmented seborrheic keratosis shows comedo-like openings and milia-like cysts

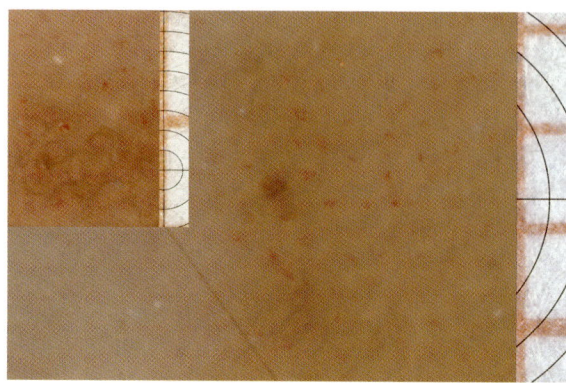

Fig. 47 Dermal nevus with vessels of the comma type

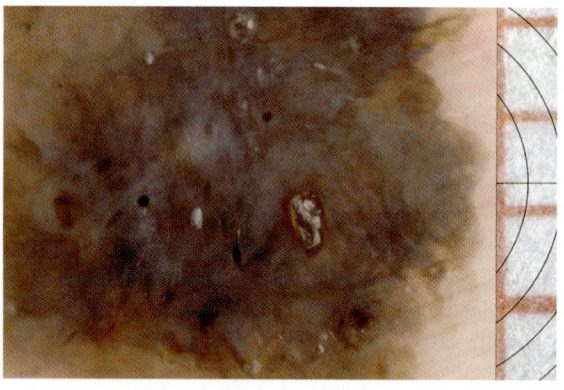

Fig. 46 Multiple comedo-like openings in the center of a fibroepithelial tumor (Pinkus)

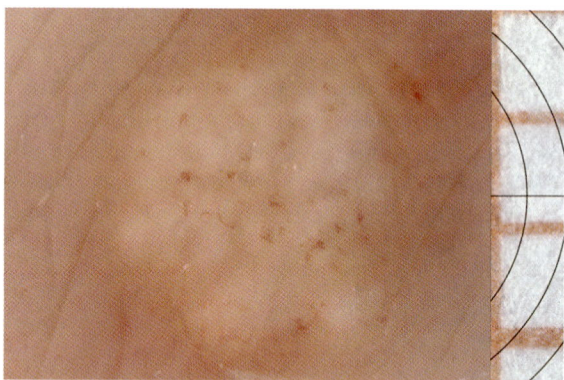

Fig. 48 Xanthoma eruptivum with a light-yellow hue shows comma-shaped vessels scattered over the surface of the tumor. The reddish corona is due to an inflammatory reaction

References

54; 63; 142; 143; 154; 184; 186; 212; 213; 221; 246; 280; 285; 316

Comma-like-shaped Vessels

Synonym

The synonym for comma-like-shaped vessels is comma vessels.

Definition

Comma-like-shaped vessels form a pattern of vascularization that consists of comma-shaped vessels that are slightly curved and running parallel to the surface of the skin.

Occurrence

Comma-like-shaped vessels occur as benign nevi, especially dermal nevi, Clark nevi, and eruptive papular xanthomas.

Surface Microscopy

Surface microscopy shows branching comma-shaped vessels which become visible as coarse and short curvilinear structures scattered over the surface of the lesion (Figs. 47, 48).

Reference

160

Compound Nevus

Synonyms
The synonyms for compound nevus are epidermal–dermal nevus and compound melanocytic nevus.

Definition
Compound nevus is a slightly elevated and sharply demarcated light- to dark-brown oval papule or nodule with a smooth or papillomatous surface.

Surface Microscopy
Surface microscopy consists of areas of regular reticular, globular, or uniform homogeneous (absent network) patterns with symmetrically distributed dots and globules, uniform in shape and size (Fig. 49). The edge is regular and fades at the periphery (gradual edge). Occasionally there are centrally hypopigmented or depigmented homogeneous areas which correspond to mature dermal melanocytes indicating loss of pigmentation. Areas of homogeneous hyperpigmentation are due to heavily pigmented keratinocytes.

Histopathology
Circumscribed nevus cell nests are located both at the dermoepidermal junction and in the papillary and reticular dermis. Melanin is found in keratinocytes, at the dermoepidermal junction, and in the superficial dermis. There may be lamellar fibrosis in the papillary dermis.

References
38; 82; 118

Congenital Hairy Nevus

▶ Congenital melanocytic nevus.

Congenital Melanocytic Nevus

Synonyms
The synonyms for congenital melanocytic nevus are congenital hairy nevus and bathing trunk nevus.

Definition
Congenital melanocytic nevus (CMN) is a melanocytic nevus that is present at birth or appears in the newborn period or months after birth. There are small (< 1.5 cm), medium (1.5–19.9 cm), and large (≥ 20 cm) lesions, but the classification of congenital nevi by size has not been based upon firm clinico-pathological-biological correlations.

Surface Microscopy
Small and medium lesions often show homogeneous patterns that consist of rete ridges with variations in shape or pigment content (Fig. 50). In some nevi the rete ridges are irregularly pigmented or distributed, which in addition to the strongly pigmented dermal nests and an increase of melanophages may result in a color of blue-gray surface hues. Large lesions are heterogeneous, displaying scattered islands of networks that are relatively symmetrical in architecture and color. The features associated with CMN include: reticular networks, globules, dots, branched streaks, diffuse pigmentation, perifollicular hypopigmentation, milia-like cysts, comedo-like openings, linear network fragments that resemble hyphal elements, and terminal hairs.

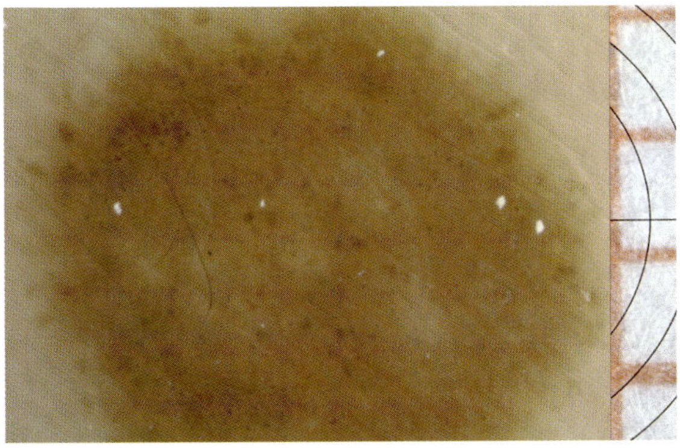

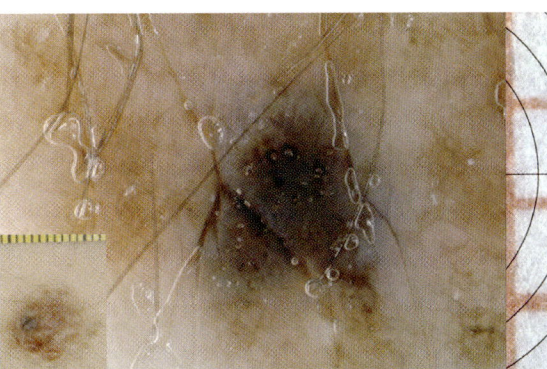

◘ **Fig. 49** Compound nevus on the upper arm is composed of symmetrically distributed globules and dots regular in size and shape

◘ **Fig. 50** Congenital melanocytic nevus associated with a malignant melanoma in situ is shown on the knee of a 28-year-old woman and consists of a fragmented pigment network and a blue-gray blotch with irregularly distributed brown dots at the periphery

Histopathology

Small lesions are characterized by melanocytes confined to the upper half of the dermis. Some melanocytes are splayed in strands between bundles of collagen far down within the reticular dermis and sometimes even in the subcutaneous fat. The nevus cells tend to be grouped around adnexal structures, nerves, blood vessels, and lymphatics. In lesions of young individuals, the melanocytes at the dermoepidermal junction frequently show variable atypia. When a melanoma develops in a congenital nevus, it usually begins to proliferate at the dermoepidermal junction.

References

5; 52; 174; 267; 268; 281

Congenital Speckled Lentiginous Nevus

▶ Nevus spilus.

Congenital Zosteriform Speckled Lentiginous Nevus

▶ Nevus spilus.

Corium

▶ Dermis.

Corneal Layer of the Epidermis

▶ Stratum corneum.

Corneocyte

Definition

Corneocyte is the dead keratin-filled squamous cell (horny cell) of the stratum corneum (horny layer).

Corticosteroid Side Effects

Chronic topical side effects of the skin depend on the duration of the use and the potency of the glucocorticosteroid employed (mild, moderate strength, potent, high potency). The typical surface microscopic features include distortion of the horny layer to form parallel striae (an early sign due to transepidermal water loss), superficial pityriasiform scaling followed by a marked epidermal thinning due to the loss of the horny layer (translucent epidermis), telangiectases and petechia develop during the inflammatory state, ostiofollicular inflammation due to immune suppression, comedones, and hypertrichosis. Atrophy of the connective tissue may occur. Corticosteroid-induced rosacea-like dermatitis present numerous yellowish lacunae, 0.5–2.0 mm in diameter, within papulovesicular or papulopustular lesions. They occur on an inflamed reddened background (dilated vasculature) and can be confluent as larger infiltrated areas. Unlike steroid acne with secondary comedones, acne rosacea is not limited to sebaceous follicles and can be quite diffuse including the interfollicular areas. Many hyperplastic follicular openings represent widened channels lined with keratinizing epithelium forming a peripheral broad brownish rim.

References

10; 39; 58; 59; 94; 99; 203; 253; 256; 299

Cotton-ball Phenomenon

▶ Psoriasis and spongiotic dermatitis.

Crista Dotted Pattern

Definition

Crista dotted pattern consists of hemoglobin-, hematoidin-, or melanin-pigmented lesions of the palms and soles showing pigmented dots and globules on the ridges (Figs. 51, 52). The ridges correspond to the crista superficialis of the skin. The openings of the eccrine ducts, which occur within the surface ridges, are spared of pigmentation.

References

110; 240

Crista Profunda Intermedia

Definition

Crista profunda intermedia consists of glabrous skin of acral areas and is characterized by the parallel arrangement of the surface skin markings referred to as dermoglyphics (parallel ridges and sulci). When the tissue sections are cut perpendicularly to the parallel

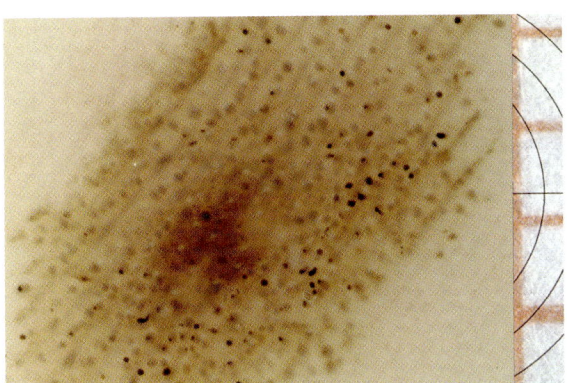

■ **Fig. 51** Crista dotted pattern of a congenital melanocytic nevus shows pigmented dots and globules on the ridges of the sole

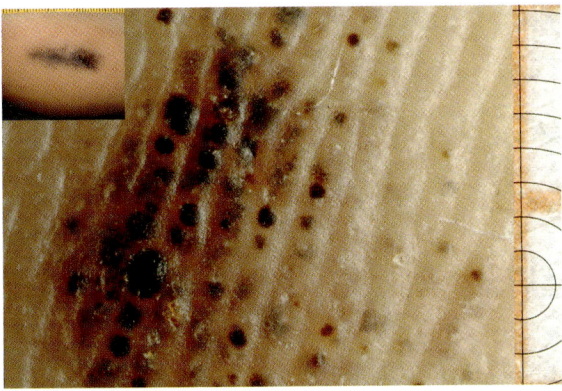

■ **Fig. 52** Black heel with a hemorrhage-induced crista dotted pattern

skin markings, the crista profunda intermedia (rete ridge) is situated under the surface ridge (crista superficialis). The rete ridge, including the crista superficialis and the crista profunda intermedia, is passed through by an intraepidermal eccrine duct (acrosyringeum). The crista profunda intermedia is where melanomas usually develop.

Reference

240

Crista Profunda Limitans

Definition

Crista profunda limitans consists of glabrous skin of acral areas and is characterized by the arrangement of parallel gyri (ridges) and sulci (furrows). When the tissue sections are cut perpendicularly to the parallel markings, the crista profunda limitans is situated un-

der the surface sulcus (furrow). The rete ridge, called crista superficialis limitans, is where nevi tend to be located.

Reference

240

Crista Reticulated Pattern

Definition

Crista reticulated pattern consists of melanocytic lesions of the palms and soles with pigmented network-like shapes. The light acrosyringium, which opens in the center of the surface ridge, is usually spared of pigmentation (Fig. 53).

References

110; 240

Crown Vessels

Definition

Crown vessels are groups of wreath-like arranged vessels located on the surface of the tumor surrounding the gland's corpus below.

Occurrence

Crown vessels occur as hyperplastic sebaceous glands.

Surface Microscopy

Surface microscopy reveals a radial arranged wreath of vessels which extend into the middle of the lesion, or a

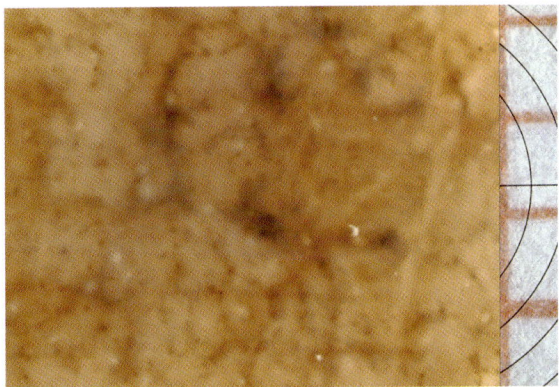

■ **Fig. 53** Crista reticulated pattern with network-like structures throughout a compound nevus of the sole

peripheral crown of regularly entwined barely branching capillaries around multiple whitish-yellow globules being filled with plugs that represent the openings of the sebaceous gland ducts (Fig. 54). The vessels may extend toward the center without arborization.

References

160; 298

Crypts

▶ Comedo-like openings.

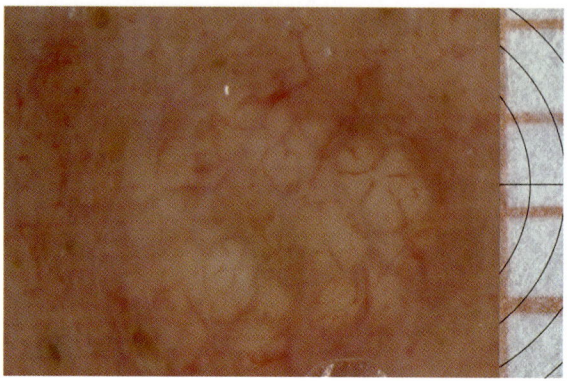

■ **Fig. 54** Sebaceous gland hyperplasia surrounded by crown vessels which extend into the middle of the nodules

Darier's Disease

Synonyms

Synonyms for Darier's disease are keratosis follicularis, Darier's disease, and dyskeratosis follicularis.

Definition

Darier's disease is an autosomal–dominant abnormality of keratinization that shows keratotic papules originating from both follicles and interfollicular epidermis. Later, papules appear crusted and verrucous.

Surface Microscopy

After removing dirty brownish keratotic plaques (acantholysis), areas of regularly arranged punctiform papillary capillaries ("naked papillae") emerge. The papillary dermis has not changed.

Histopathology

Focal suprabasal acantholytic dyskeratosis and lacunae in the slightly acanthotic epidermis as well as hyperkeratosis and patchy parakeratosis are typical signs. Eosinophilic dyskeratotic cells with premature cornification (corps ronds and grains) issue in the epidermis.

References

2; 58; 226

Degenerative Changes with Blue-gray Granules in the Marginal Area

► Regression pattern.

Dendritic Grayish-blue Trabeculae

► Trabeculae of melanophages.

Depigmentation

Definition

Absence of visible pigment in a pigmented skin lesion. The depigmented region has less pigmentation than background skin. In benign lesions depigmentation is a common change and usually found in the center. Depigmentation may indicate histopathological changes of regression in pigmented lesions (regression pattern), or it may be found in the dermal component as a result of the absence of pigmented cells. In melanomas and amelanotic nodules of melanoma depigmentation is irregularly localized at any site of the lesion and it is often found near the border. Irregular depigmentation has a specificity of 92% and a sensitivity 46% for invasive melanoma.

References

82; 184; 200; 204; 205; 286

Dermal Nevus

Synonym

The synonym for dermal nevus is intradermal melanocytic nevus.

Definition

Skin-colored to light-brown sharply demarcated oval papule or nodule (5–10 mm in diameter) which is formed entirely by nevus cells in the dermis. The lesion may have a papillomatous surface.

Surface Microscopy

Dermal nevi generally have an symmetric slight pigmented globular, papillomatous cobblestone or homogeneous pattern (Fig. 55). Due to their loss of the junctional components, they may be relatively struc-

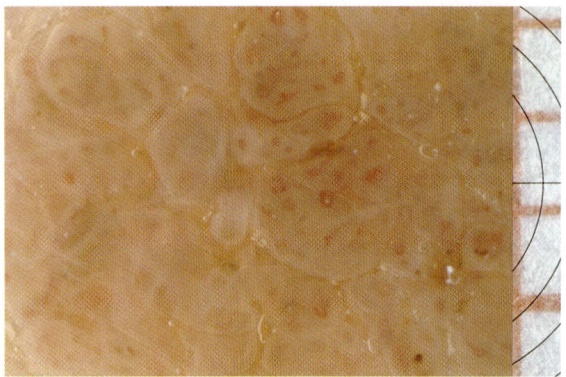

▪ Fig. 55 Dermal nevus on the trunk shows a light-brown pigmented cobblestone pattern and comma- or hairpin-like-shaped vessels

tureless, amelanotic and homogeneous, or they present with a less developed pigment network and black dots. In facial lesions a pseudonetwork can be seen. Though relatively avascular, individual comma- and/or hairpin-like-shaped blood vessels are frequently found.

Histopathology

In the dermis there are nests and strands of melanocytes. In the deeper part the melanocytes are smaller and may become spindle shaped (neurotization) with little or no pigment.

References
38; 82; 118

Dermal Papilla

Definition
Papillae of the connective tissue (stratum papillare of the dermis) interdigitate with the rete ridges in the overlying epidermis. From the superficial dermal plexus the terminal capillary loops extend to supply each individual papillae.

Surface Microscopy
The papillae contain vascular loops of 0.01–0.02 mm in diameter. In the skin surface red dots indicate the center of the papillae. A thick horny layer of the epidermis obscures the red dots. The pigment network is a lace-like pattern, which is the result of the rete ridges (constituting the trabeculae) and areas of less dense

pigmentation, which are due to the dermal papillae (constituting the holes of the network; Fig. 56).

References
58; 160; 262; 284

Dermatitis Herpetiformis Duhring

▸ Marks sign.

Dermatofibroma

Synonyms
Synonyms for dermatofibroma are histiocytoma, fibroma durum, and hard fibroma.

Definition
Benign hard dermal nodule with a yellowish to reddish-brown dome-shaped surface that characteristically dimple (distinct pinch sign, or "button hole") when pressed at the edges.

Surface Microscopy
Dermatofibroma most commonly presents with a sharply demarcated central white, scar-like patch with a surrounding pigmented network and/or brown pigmentation (Fig. 57). The network corresponds to long, regularly distributed and heavily pigmented rete ridges. The scar-like area often contains brown globule-like

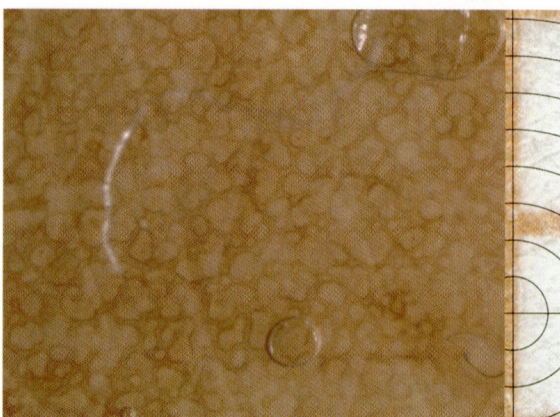

▪ Fig. 56 Normal well-pigmented skin on the dorsum. The "holes" of the pigmented network (areas of little pigment) are due to the dermal papillae. In addition, some hardly visible point-like vessels, representing the terminal capillaries, indicate the site of the papillae

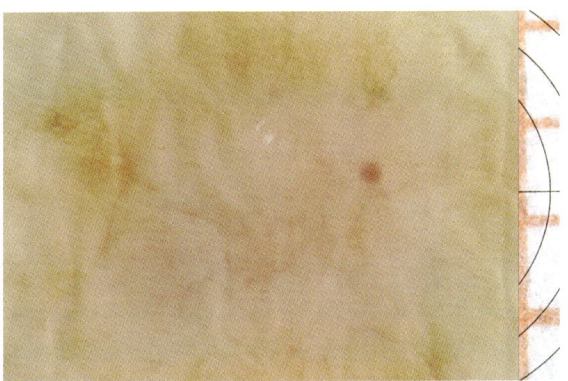

Fig. 57 Dermatofibroma on the lower leg demonstrates a central whitish-reddish scar-like area and a surrounding peripheral network due to hyperpigmented rete ridges

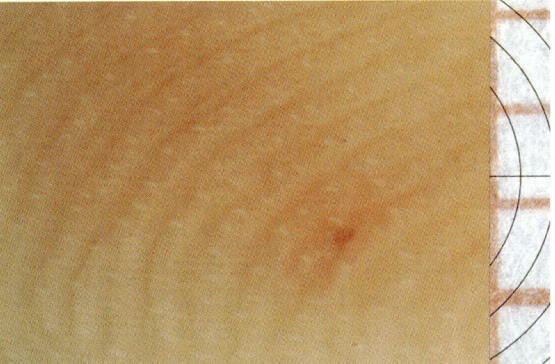

Fig. 58 Parallel gyri (ridges) form arches and sulci (furrows) of the fingertip. The eccrine ducts are arranged regularly in the center of the ridges

structures (due to pigmented flat and confluent rete ridges) and occasionally contains blood vessels.

Histopathology

The tumor is composed of areas of fibroblasts and interwoven (storiform) collagen fiber bundles without elastic fibers. The overlying epidermis may be hyperplastic and show basal cell carcinoma-like structures.

References

58; 68; 77; 96; 137; 188

Dermatoglyphics

Definition

Dermatoglyphics represent the configuration of the parallel ridges and furrows of the volar skin surface. In the human hand, the distal segment of each digit has three types of configurations: whorl; loop; and arch.

Surface Microscopy

Openings of eccrine ducts are seen as whitish dots regularly arranged in the center of the ridges with a space of 0.4–0.5 mm (Fig. 58). The diameter of a nonpigmented dot (acrosyringium), including a whitish halo, takes 0.08 mm. Diameters of the ostia vary between 0.02 and 0.04 mm.

Histopathology

The ridges correspond to the crista superficialis and the furrows correspond to the sulcus superficialis. Openings of the eccrine duct occur within the surface ridge.

References

110; 240; 262; 284

Dermatomyositis

▶ Nailfold capillaries, alterations.

Dermis

Synonyms

Synonyms for the dermis are corium and cutis vera.

Definition

A layer of skin composed of a superficial thin layer that interdigitates with the epidermis (dermal papillae and rete ridges), the stratum papillare, and the stratum reticulare. The dermal tissue consists of a network of collagen and elastic fibers that are embedded in a mucopolysaccharide ground substance matrix. The cellular components are fibroblasts which produce the ground substance and fibers, as well as macrophages and mast cells. In addition, the dermis contains blood and lymphatic vessels, nerves and nerve endings, glands, and, except for glabrous skin, hair follicles.

Desmoplastic Melanoma

Definition

Desmoplastic melanoma is a malignant melanocytic lesion that represents mainly a red, grayish, or brown macule with irregular demarcation or a firm flat papule (fibroma-like; Fig. 59), and it may be a predominantly amelanotic lesion. The tumor consists of atypical spindle-shaped cells with an increased dermal connective tissue component.

Surface Microscopy

Characteristic melanoma features are absent in most cases. In initial stages there may be an inconspicuous grayish macule or papule with a hypopigmented center. Follow-up examinations of the lesion reveal asymmetric growth, border irregularity, and color variability. Photoaging and intense skin atrophy can cause a complete effacement of the pseudonetwork on facial regions. Subtle grayish patches, grayish-brown amorphous blotches, and capillary loop enlargement, as well as teleangiectasia and tortuous dilated vessels, can be seen at the periphery and/or in the center of the lesion. In addition, some capillaries are accompanied by clusters of small blue-gray punctuated particles (melanophages).

Histopathology

There is the subtle proliferation of melanocytes presenting as solitary units or as small nests at the dermoepidermal junction. The atypical, spindle-shaped melanocytes are arranged in fascicles, intermingled with fibrillary collagen bundles. The neoplastic wavy melanocytes may form structures that resemble authentic nerve fascicles (neurotropic melanoma). There are moderately dense lymphocytic aggregates associated with the neoplastic proliferation.

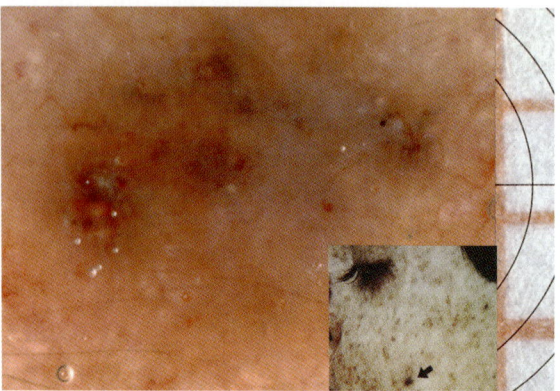

Fig. 59 Asymmetric, irregularly bordered desmoplastic melanoma (Clark level IV, Breslow thickness 1.68 mm) on the cheek, measuring 3.5 mm in maximal diameter, with unstructured aggregates of grayish pigment concentrations surrounded by a light-brown haze (*inset, arrow*), in an 11-year-old boy with xeroderma pigmentosum

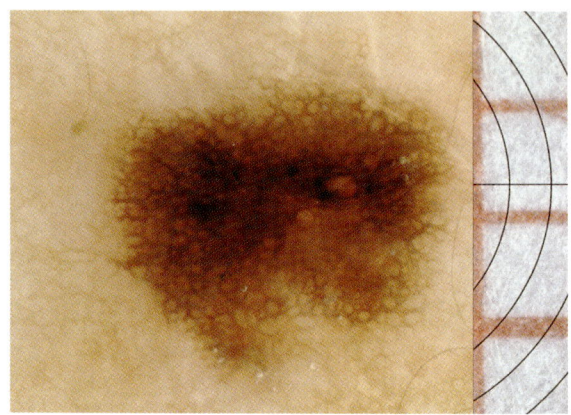

Fig. 60 Junctional nevus with a diffuse network pattern

References

5; 13; 36; 73; 87; 127; 152; 229; 230; 259; 262; 275

Desmoplastic Spitz Nevus

► Irregular vessels.

Diffuse Network Pattern

Definition

The diffuse network pattern is a melanocytic lesion with a uniformly prominent pigmented network throughout the tumor.

Occurrence

Diffuse network pattern occurs as lentigines, benign nevi, and clinically atypical nevi.

Surface Microscopy

The light-brown to dark-brown network lines are generally thin, uniform, and discrete, and fade at the periphery of the lesion (Fig. 60).

Reference

304

Diffuse Network with Central Globules

Synonym

The synonym for diffuse network with central globules is reticulo-globular pattern.

Definition

Melanocytic nevus representing a peripheral network pattern with regularly located central globules (Fig. 61) is indicative of a benign nature of the lesion.

Reference

304

Diffuse Pigmentation

Synonyms

Synonyms for diffuse pigmentation are diffuse multi-component pigmentation, diffuse pigmentation with variable shades, diffuse background pigmentation, and irregular diffuse pigmentation.

Definition

Diffuse pigmentation is a melanocytic lesion with irregular diffuse distribution of brown to black background pigment.

Occurrence

Diffuse pigmentation occurs as malignant melanomas and congenital melanocytic nevi.

Surface Microscopy

When the rete ridges are poorly defined and flat, no pigment network is seen. The structureless diffuse background pigmentation is brown with variable shades from tan to black (epidermal or dermal pigment; Fig. 62) but is occasionally accompanied by a bluish gray tone.

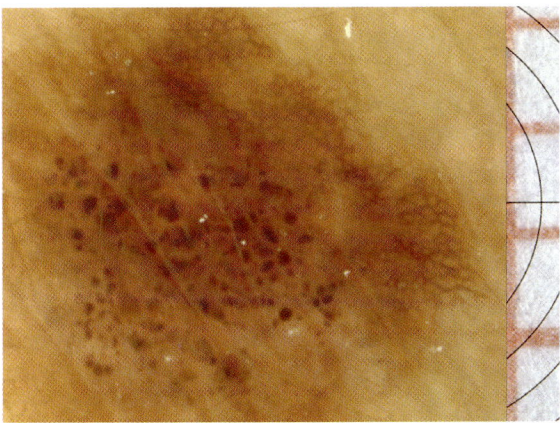

◻ Fig. 61 Compound nevus with a peripheral network pattern and central globules

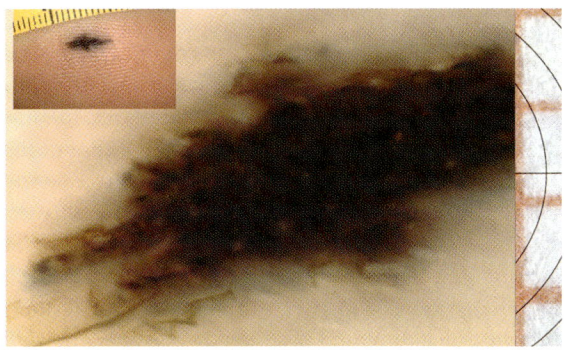

◻ Fig. 62 Congenital junctional melanocytic nevus on the heel. Diffuse pigmentation throughout the lesion with variable shades from brown to black, accompanied by a bluish gray tone at the bottom side of the border, is seen

References

140; 143; 174; 239; 240

Digitiform Extrusions

▸ Radial streaming.

Discoid Lupus Erythematosus

▸ Tack phenomenon.
▸ Autoimmunogenic keratinocytolysis.

Dots

Synonyms

Synonyms for dots are black dots, brown dots, and brown/black dots on a blue-gray background.

Definition

Dots are round or oval structures of less than 0.1 mm in diameter that may be black, dark brown, gray, or blue-gray (due to the level of pigment in the skin) within pigmented lesions. They represent localized pigment accumulation in the horny layer, or less often in the deeper aspects of the epidermis.

Occurrence

Dots occur as benign (regular in size and distribution), dysplastic and malignant melanocytic lesions (irregular, mostly at or near the edge of the lesion), and pigmented basal cell carcinoma.

Surface Microscopy

In benign lesions, black/brown dots tend to be central in position and are regular in size, shape, and distribution (Figs. 63, 64). In malignant or dysplastic lesions, they also occur in the periphery or near the edge of the lesion, vary in size and shape, and they are irregularly distributed and mainly localized on a blue-gray background. Multiple brown dots are highly significant feature of invasive melanoma, in contrast to scattered or isolated brown dots seen in many benign lesions. Multiple blue-gray dots are seen as partly aggregated dots (melanophages) in association with a regression pattern.

Histopathology

The color of the dots is determined by the level of pigment in the skin. Black dots represent localized

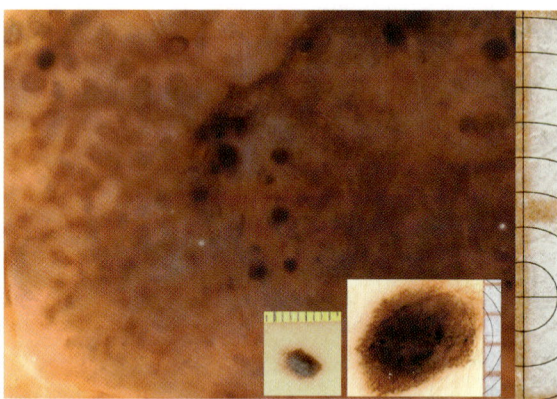

■ **Fig. 63** Compound nevus with some black and blue-gray dots in the center of the lesion

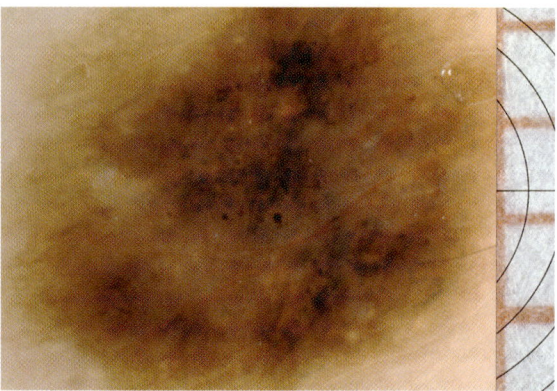

■ **Fig. 64** Superficial spreading melanoma in the scapular region (Clark level III, Breslow thickness 0.65 mm). Irregularly distributed black dots varying in size are shown

pigment accumulation often due to melanoma cells in the stratum corneum and in the upper part of the epidermis. Brown dots are due to suprabasal (intraepidermal) collections of pigment or focal melanin accumulation (pigmented cell nests) at the dermoepidermal junction. Blue-gray, blue, or purple granules (peppering) represent melanin-laden macrophages, loose melanin, fine melanin particles (melanin "dust") in melanophages, or free melanin in the deep papillary or reticular dermis.

References
21; 46; 82; 111; 142; 143; 186; 188; 200; 211; 212; 213; 222; 279; 280; 298

Dotted Vessels

Synonym

The synonym for dotted vessels is pinpoint vessels.

Definition

Dotted vessels are tiny red dot-like short vessels (< 0.1 mm in diameter) within the amelanotic component or throughout a melanocytic or non-melanocytic lesion.

Occurrence

Dotted vessels occur as malignant melanoma (within amelanotic or hypomelanotic components), Clark nevi, Spitz nevi, Bowen's disease, psoriasis, and dermatitis.

Surface Microscopy

Surface microscopy shows regularly arranged pinpoint-like vessels (0.01–0.02 mm in diameter) densely aligned next to each other representing the terminal capillaries of the dermal papillae. They are seen as circumscribed zones within a regressive hypomelanotic area of melanoma (Figs. 65, 66). They may also occur by forming a regularly arranged base pattern throughout the entire lesion, within epithelial tumors or erythemato-squamous skin diseases throughout the lesion.

Reference
160

Drug-induced Hyperpigmentation

▶ Hyperpigmentation.

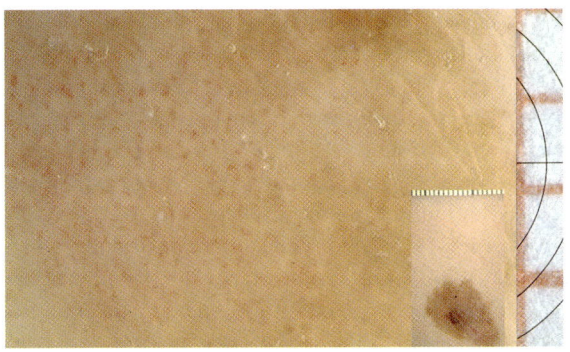

Fig. 65 Superficial spreading melanoma (Clark level II, Breslow thickness 0.56 mm) on the forearm with an area of extensive pinpoint (dotted) vessels in the amelanotic component

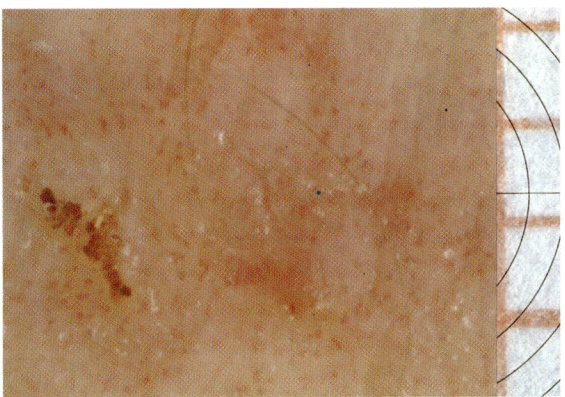

Fig. 66 Bowen's disease of the back of the hand shows dotted vessels throughout the lesion

Dyskeratosis

Definition
Dyskeratosis is premature keratinization in individual keratinocytes that have not yet reached the upper layers of the epidermis, corps ronds, or hyaline cells, and clumping of cells. Some cells have become apoptotic.

References
262; 287

Dyskeratosis Follicularis

▸ Darier's disease.

Dyskeratosis Maligna

▸ Bowen's disease.

Dysplastic Nevi, Basic Patterns

Definition
Dysplastic nevi can be classified into 12 categories (Table 3).

Reference
122

Dysplastic Nevi, ELM Rating Protocol

Definition
The ELM Rating Protocol is a system designed to differentiate nevocellular nevi from dysplastic/atypical nevi by assigning a point score to the findings on epi-

Table 3 Basic patterns of dysplastic nevi. (Modified according to [122])

Pattern	Assessment
Reticular	Suggests benign lesion
Globular	Typical benign cobblestone architecture
Homogeneous	Suggests benign lesion
Reticular–globular	Suggests benign lesion
Reticular–homogeneous	Suggests benign lesion
Homogeneous–globular	Suggests benign lesion
Central hyperpigmented	Suggests benign lesion
Central hypopigmented	Suggests benign lesion
Peripheral hypopigmented	Requires excision or close follow-up
Eccentric hyperpigmented	Requires excision or close follow-up
Multifocal hyper-/hypopigmented	Requires excision or close follow-up
Unclassified	Requires excision or close follow-up

luminescent microscopic (surface microscopic) examination (Table 4).

References

13; 255; 258

Dysplastic Nevus

Synonyms

Synonyms for dysplastic nevus are atypical nevus, Clark's nevus, and melanocytic nevus with irregular architecture.

Definition

Dysplastic nevi are flat or slightly elevated benign melanocytic lesions showing an uneven border and an asymmetric pigmentation pattern with varying shades of pigment (ranging from light tan to brown mixed with pink and black hues). Histology may reveal cytological atypism of junctional melanocytes in association with architectural disorder. They have been shown to serve as markers for an increased risk of developing melanoma, and they are considered to be precursor lesions to melanoma, especially when associated with the familiar type of dysplastic nevus syndrome. At the present time, there is no uniform agreement about what a dysplastic nevus is, because the terms "dysplasia" or "dysplastic nevi" have not yet been defined histopathologically and cytobiologically in a repeatable, comprehensible way; therefore, some authors recommend to abolish the designations of architectural and cytological irregularities in melanocytic nevi and prefer the eponym of Clark's nevus.

Surface Microscopy

Dysplastic nevi may possess many features which are commonly seen in melanoma. They often have an irregular reticular or multicomponent pattern. Irregular pigmentation stops often abruptly at the periphery. The pigment network is focally prominent and atypical. Irregular dots and globules of varying shapes, sizes, and distribution can be seen throughout the lesion (Fig. 67). Reddish or pink macular or papular components, as well as melanin "dust," blue-gray veils or regression structures (melanin peppering) with diffuse depigmentation, or hypopigmentation may be found. Radial streaming and pseudopods are absent

◘ Table 4 Epiluminescent microscopic rating protocol for dysplastic nevocellular nevi

Characteristic	Point value
Black dot on blue background	10
Area with evenly arranged capillaries	10
Pseudopod-like structure of the margin	10
Degenerative changes with blue-gray granules in the marginal area	9
Abrupt loss of pigment in the trabeculae	7
Dendritic grayish-blue trabeculae (streaks of melanophages)	6
Bizarre reticular pattern	5
Multicomponent pattern	5
Gray color tone	2
Grayish-blue globules in the center of the papillae	2

Evaluation: Point total 10–15 = suspicious of dysplasia (may be melanoma); point total > 15 = suspicious of high-grade dysplasia (suggest melanoma)

The specific histopathological criteria of dysplastic/atypical nevi are still debated. The diagnosis is therefore based on a combination of clinical and histological evaluation; thus, if the histological diagnosis were "dysplastic" or "atypical" nevus and the preoperative surface microscopic image analysis indicates 15 or more total points, there would be a very high suspicion of malignancy

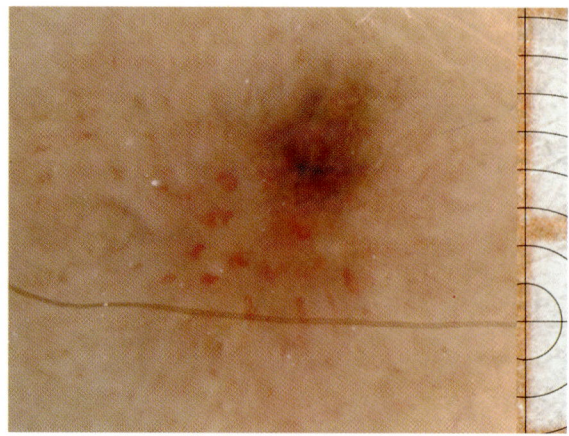

◘ Fig. 67 Dysplastic nevus with a corona of small punctiform vessels on a light-brown background, an area of irregular vessels and an area of gray blotches, shows a typical multicomponent pattern

features (e.g., dysplastic or atypical nevi, dermoscopic properties; Table 5).

Histopathology

The epidermis tends to have elongation of the rete ridges with proliferation of normal or variable atypical melanocytes either singly or in nests at the dermoepidermal junction. All of the melanocytes are situated at the dermoepidermal junction and not far above it. The irregularly distributed nests often show bridging between two rete ridges. There are also an increased number of melanocytes at the periphery of the lesion beyond the area of the dermal component (shoulder phenomenon). The dermis shows lamellar and concentric eosinophilic fibroplasia, lymphocytic infiltrates, and pigment incontinence.

References

3; 6; 7; 8; 11; 13; 14; 33; 64; 70; 71; 82; 103; 108; 109; 112; 114; 118; 147; 149; 166; 201; 242; 248; 250; 274; 287; 298; 303

Dysplastic or Atypical Nevi, Dermoscopic Properties

Definition

Atypical or dysplastic nevi are melanocytic nevi with cytological atypia of junctional melanocyte/nevus cells in association with architectural atypia.

Reference

107

◘ **Table 5** Dermoscopic properties of dysplastic or atypical nevi. (Adapted from [186, 303])

Commonly present	Occasionally present	Typically not present
Asymmetrical pigmentation pattern	Symmetrical pigmentation pattern	Peripheral black dots
Irregular, discrete pigment network	Irregular, prominent pigment network	Pseudopods
Irregularly distributed and shaped	Irregular depigmentation	Radial streaming brown globules
Pigment network that fades gradually at the periphery	Pigment network that ends abruptly at the periphery	Blue-white veil
		Homogeneous areas (more than 25% of the total area) and five or more of the following colors: red; blue; black; tan; gray; dark brown

Eccentric Hyperpigmented Pattern

Definition

Eccentric hyperpigmented pattern consists of a melanocytic lesion representing an irregular eccentric hyperpigmented area which may be brown to slate-gray in color (Fig. 68). That alteration of pigmentation suggests dysplastic and/or malignant changes and requires either close follow-up or excision.

Eccrine Pores

Definition

Eccrine pores are openings of eccrine ducts. Eccrine sweat glands (glandulae sudoriferae) are involved primarily in the thermoregulation and are spread over the entire body.

Surface Microscopy

Eccrine pores are recognized as whitish dots. If the opening of the duct has a slit-type aperture, it may be invisible. Diameter of the ostia vary between 0.02 and 0.04 mm. A whitish halo surrounding the acrosyringium takes 0.08 mm in diameter. Acral skin of the palms and soles is characterized by a parallel ridge pattern composed of ridges (crista superficialis) and furrows (sulcus superficialis). The openings of the eccrine ducts are regularly arranged in the center of the papillary ridges with a space of 0.4–0.5 mm. The intraepithelial section of the epidermal duct (acrosyringium) is pigment-free and twisted in the fashion of a corkscrew (Figs. 69, 70).

References

110; 240

Ehring's Rhexis Bleeding

▶ Nailfold capillaries, changes.

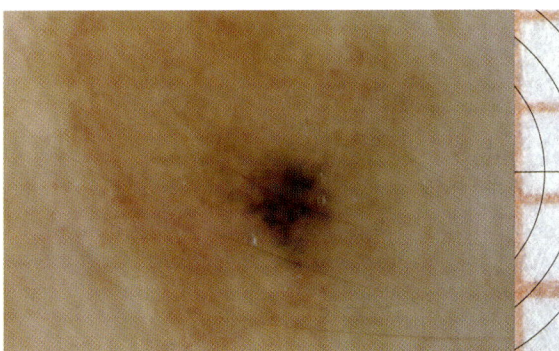

■ **Fig. 68** Dysplastic compound nevus on the back shows an eccentric slate-gray area

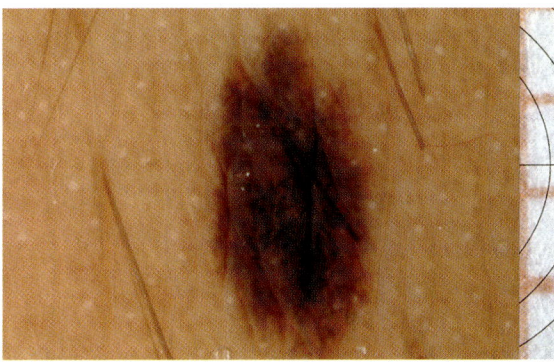

■ **Fig. 69** Ultraviolet-induced pigmentation in the umbilical region with regularly distributed pigment-free light dots represents openings of eccrine ducts, and in addition, there is a compound nevus

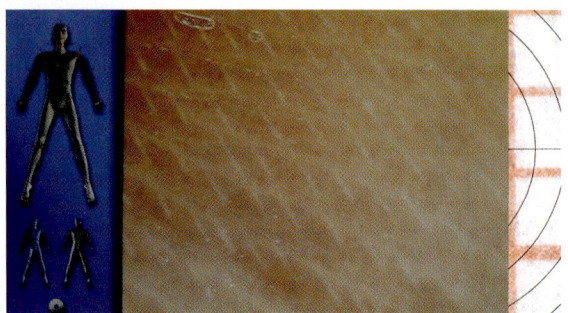

Fig. 70 Corksrew-like twisted acrosyringia of the sole

Elastosis

Degenerative changes in elastic tissue (e.g., actinic elastosis) indicate an increase in connective tissue fibers in the dermis associated with a destruction of the subepithelial elastic plexus. Below the narrow band of elastica-free connective tissue there is a concentration of thickened, amorphous, fibrillar, or plaque-like material, with the histological staining characteristics of elastic fibers. On surface microscopy finely striated, or diffuse, structureless ivory or yellowish plaques under the thinned atrophic epidermis are frequently visible. Additional typical associated features are as follows: abnormal follicular keratinization; regression of the epidermal ridges; prominent capillary loops; dilated and aneurysmal vessels of the subpapillary plexus; and pigmentary incontinency.

ELM Grading Protocol

Definition

The ELM Grading Protocol classifies the epiluminescence microscopy (surface microscopy) features for the diagnosis of malignant melanoma. A melanocytic lesion should be considered as malignant if two or more of the listed criteria are present (see Table 6).

References

36; 143

Enhanced ABCD-E Scoring System

Definition

The enhanced ABCD-E scoring system is calculated by adding 1.2 to a lesion's standard ABCD score for patient-noted changes of a melanocytic lesion and by subtracting 0.8 for non-changing lesions. The standard and enhanced scoring systems are given in Tables 7 and 8, respectively.

Reference

174

Table 6 The ELM grading protocol to diagnose malignant melanoma. (Modified from [143])
Multicomponent pattern (three or more different ELM appearances)
Nodular pattern (one or more regions of irregular, dark, dense pigment concentration)
Pseudopods (irregular finger-like projections of dark pigment at the periphery)
Radial streaming (irregular radial extensions of pigment at the periphery)
Irregular extensions (may appear within a lesion and may be much larger than pseudopods)
Whitish veil or milky way (ground-glass-appearing haze or veil over a region of the lesion)
Blue-gray veil (appearing over a peppering of very small black particles)
Peripheral pigment dots (punctate pigment that may be black, nearly black or dark brown)
Capillary prominence (small capillaries appearing to be neovascularization)
Capillary dot pattern (a cluster of capillaries appear as a region of red dots)
Network irregularity (average overall irregularity of the pigment network)
Abrupt cut-off of the network (abrupt transition in pigmentation)
High-order network branching (tree-like thick network lines that branch into pseudopods)
Peripheral dark network patches (relatively darker network lines than the average network)
Variability of the thickness of the network lines

Table 7 Standard ABCD scoring system

	Possible score	No. of choices for each criterion (range)	Description	Weight factor (range)
Asymmetry (assess contour, colors, structures)	0: symmetry in both axes	0–2 (A)	×1.3	0–2.6
	1: asymmetry in one axis			
	2: asymmetry in both axes			
Border	0–8: number of border segments with abrupt cut-off of pigment pattern	0–8 (B)	×0.1	0–0.8
Color	1–6: number of colors present within the lesion	1–6 (C)	×0.5	0.5–3
	White			
	Red			
	Light brown			
	Dark brown			
	Blue-gray			
	Black			
Dermoscopic structure	1–5: number of dermoscopic structures	1–5 (D)	×0.5	0.5–2.5
	Pigment network			
	Structureless area			
	Dots			
	Globules			
	Streaks			

Total possible combined score: $[(A \times 1.3) + (B \times 0.1) + (C \times 0.5) + (D \times 0.5)] = 1.0\text{–}8.9$

Table 8 Enhanced ABCD-E score. (Adapted from [173])

Criteria	Score
Asymmetry, **B**order, **C**olor and **D**ermoscopic structure	Standard ABCD score
Enlargement or other morphological changes as reported by the patient	+1.2 for a changing lesion
	−0.8 for a non-changing lesion
Total enhanced ABCD-E score =	
Standard ABCD score + 1.2 for changing lesion	
Standard ABCD score −0.8 for a non-changing lesion	

Ephelis

Synonym

The synonym for ephelis is freckle.

Definition

An ephelis is a uniform hyperpigmented solar-induced flat macule that has an increase of melanin in the basal keratinocytes and a normal number of melanocytes. They typically fade in the winter months.

Surface Microscopy

A typical feature is the moth-eaten border. The uniform pigmented background color varies from yellow to yellow-brown or dark brown, depending on sun exposure. Brown globules are absent and no pigmented network is seen.

Reference

188

Epitheloid Cell Nevus

▶ Spitz nevus.

Eruptive Hemangioma

▶ Hemangiomas.

Erythema

Synonym

The synonym for erythema is capillary prominence.

Definition

Erythema refers to hemoglobin reflectance of mildly dilated central capillary loops within the dermal papillae or of dilated linear, horizontal, and/or tortuous vessels (telangiectasia) of the subepidermal plexus. It is seen mainly within areas of regression, at the border of the lesion or in zones of neovascularization.

Reference

143

Facial Skin

Surface Microscopy

The anatomy of facial skin differs from that of non-facial zones in that the rete ridges, especially in elderly persons and UV-light-damaged integument, are much more diminished than in other regions, with the exception of well-pigmented younger or black skin (Fig. 71). In some cases the facial rete ridges may be absent. In addition, adnexal structures are more prominent and greater in number on the face; thus, a typical pigment network with the regular honeycomb pattern is rarely found on adult facial skin. Instead, a rough reticular pattern called pseudonetwork with a broad mesh and light holes is created by numerous pigment-free terminal and vellus hair follicles (Fig. 72), as well as sweat glands ostia. Small red dots corresponding with the terminal capillaries in the center of the dermal papillae are rare to absent.

References

246; 271

Fibrillar Pattern

Synonym

The synonym for fibrillar pattern is filamentous pattern.

Definition

Fibrillar pattern is a melanocytic lesion on acral volar or plantar skin with mesh-like or filamentous, densely arranged fibrillar pigmentation crossing the lines of skin markings.

Occurrence

Fibrillar pattern consists of usually benign volar and plantar nevi, and sometimes malignant melanocytic lesions.

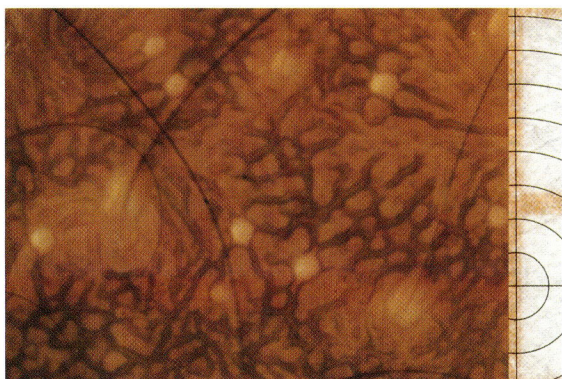

Fig. 71 Normal forehead skin of a young black African shows a pigmented network, evenly shaped light openings of eccrine ducts, and two openings of vellus hair follicles

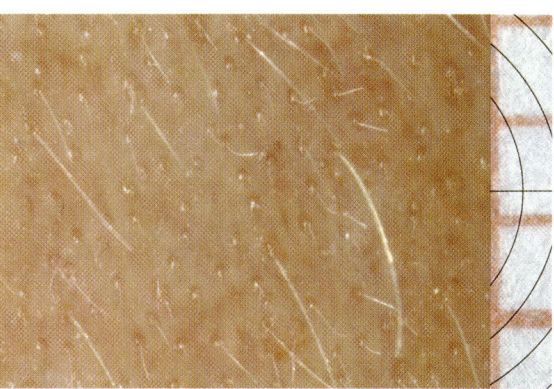

Fig. 72 Central facial skin of a young white woman shows vellus hair follicles and a lack of pigmented network

Surface Microscopy

Surface microscopy shows densely packed, finely pigmented parallel filaments that cross the furrows (sulcus superficialis) in a slanted direction (Fig. 73).

Histopathology

Melanin granules are distributed along an oblique arrangement of the epidermis and particularly of the cornified layer.

References

207; 238; 240

Fibrosis

Definition

Fibrosis is formation of fibrous tissue as a reparative or reactive process. In replacement the fibrous tissue occupies the sites of various other cells, e.g., melanoma cells, with subsequent tissue atrophy, degeneration, and necrosis.

Surface Microscopy

Fibrosis is responsible for the white color (depigmentation of the skin) seen under surface micoscopy.

Reference

44

Fingerprint-like Structures

Synonym

The synonym for fingerprint-like structures is fingerprint-like pattern.

Definition

Fingerprint-like structures are tiny light-brown ridges of pigmented lesions running in parallel and producing a pattern that resembles fingerprints.

Occurrence

Fingerprint-like structures occur as flat seborrheic keratoses and solar lentigo.

Surface Microscopy

The fine, compact light-brown cords (network lines; Fig. 74) are loose and linearly striated, giving a fingerprint-like appearance. The overall pattern shows loose net-like structures rather than a distinct pigment network.

References

55; 142; 245; 280; 298; 316

Fissures and Ridges

Synonyms

The synonyms for fissures and ridges are brain-like appearance, gyri and sulci, cerebriform appearance, and mountain and valley pattern.

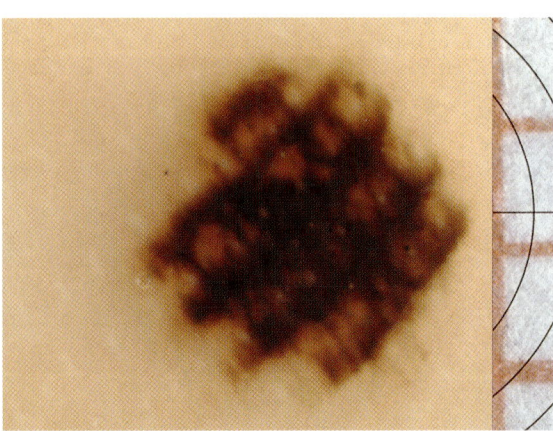

Fig. 73 Combination of the fibrillar pattern, thick filamentous variant, and the parallel furrow pattern in a junctional nevus of the sole

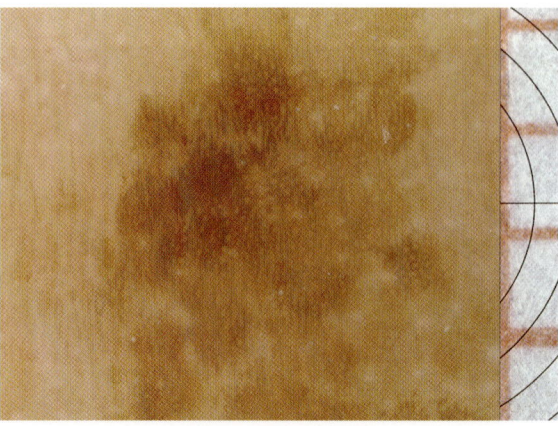

Fig. 74 Solar lentigo shows a fingerprint-like pattern. There are many linear and striated network lines arranged parallel to each other

Definition

Multiple deep furrows or clefts (fissures) and crests (ridges) in a pigmented lesion much looking like a mountain and valley pattern or the surface of the brain.

Occurrence

Acanthotic seborrheic keratoses, congenital melanocytic nevi, papillomatous dermal and compound nevi.

Surface Microscopy

Fissures are light to dark brown or black linear depressions forming confluent and branching sulci and gyri within the lesion. Ridges are linear lightly pigmented elevations on the surface of the lesion (Fig. 75).

Histopathology

Wedge-shaped clefts and deep invaginations of the epidermis filled with keratin of the stratum corneum.

References

21; 55; 142; 245; 280; 316

Follicular Plug and Opening

Definition

The pilosebaceous unit is composed of a hair follicle, a sebaceous gland that is attached to it, and the products of these structures, e.g., keratinized material, cellular membrane structures, and sebum. There are three different types of follicles in human skin: terminal hair follicle; vellus hair follicle; and sebaceous gland follicles (characteristic of human beings and not present in animals). Huge sebaceous gland follicles are found on the face and the central parts of chest and back. They have a large orifice (up to 0.45 mm in diameter) and generally contain a very small, sometimes rudimentary, hair. The surrounding connective tissue (stratum papillare) include evenly arranged punctiform capillary loops (originally from the superficial dermal plexus), supplying the papillae. In the center of the face the number of sebaceous gland follicles and vellus hair follicles range from 450 to 850/cm². The diameters of the follicle ostia vary between 0.09 and 0.45 mm.

Surface Microscopy

On surface microscopy the hair and sebaceous gland follicles are seen as well-defined round "target" structures, i.e., target-like (targetoid) pattern (Figs. 76, 77). The tan-to-brown central plug is surrounded by a yellowish-whitish-opaque circular rim corresponding to the inner root sheath (i.e., granular layer), a broader

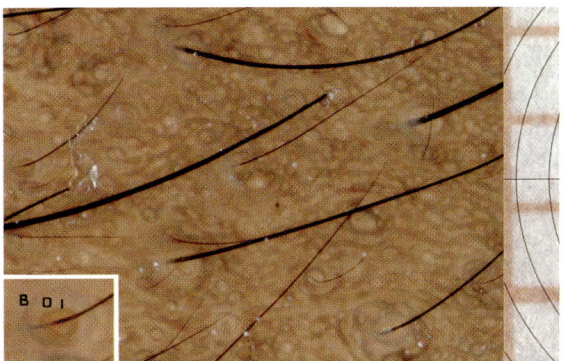

Fig. 76 Follicular openings (vellus hair and sebaceous gland follicles) on an intense pigmented central facial skin of a young man (targetoid pattern: *I* inner-root sheath; *O* outer-root sheath; *B* basal lamina)

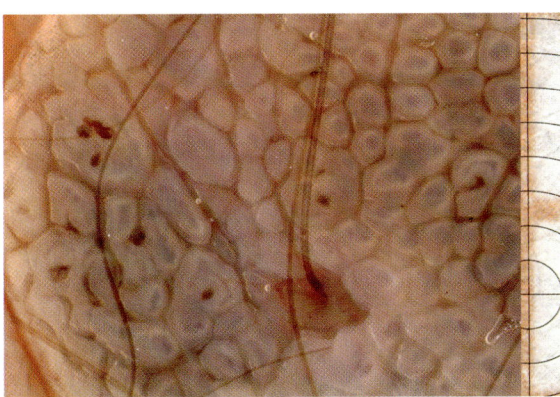

Fig. 75 Seborrheic keratosis on the neck represents fissures and ridges in a cerebriform (brain-like) appearance

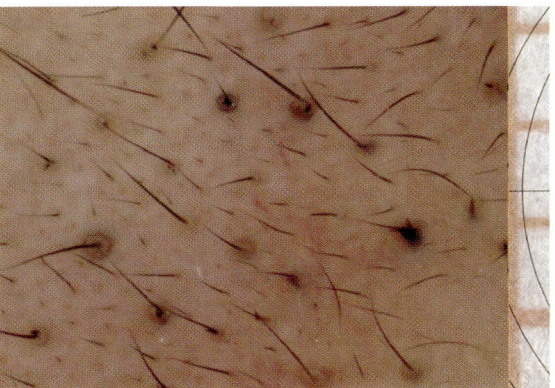

Fig. 77 Follicular openings (vellus hair follicles) in a poor pigmented perinasal region of a young woman with black hairs

and more transparent ring corresponding to the outer root sheath (i.e., spinous layer), and the outermost more or less melanin-pigmented thinner circular basal lamina. Asymmetric pigmented follicular openings correspond to the dark pigmentation in an asymmetric distribution due to the different depths of concentrated atypical melanocytes within the basal layer of individual hair follicles (perifollicular pigment changes).

References

121; 184; 188; 245; 262

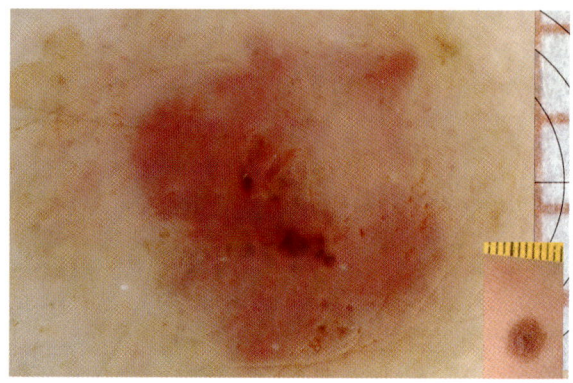

◨ **Fig. 78** Irritated compound nevus represents a fried-egg pattern with a hemorrhage in the center of the lesion

Fried-egg Pattern

Definition

Melanocytic lesion with a hemorrhage or a black lamella (parakeratotic scale containing melanin) in the center.

Surface Microscopy

In irritated melanocytic nevi there may be a hemorrhagic scale and crust in the center (Fig. 78). Pattern variations in the center, e.g., hyper- or hypopigmentation, globules, dots, branched streaks, can be indicative of malignant growth.

Reference

298

Gray-blue Areas

► GBA.
► Blue-white veil.

Globular Pattern

Definition

Globular pattern consists of melanocytic lesions with numerous round-to-oval structures, usually larger than 0.1 mm in diameter.

Occurrence

Globular pattern occurs as benign nevi (globules are uniform and regular distributed), Spitz nevi, malignant melanoma, and dysplastic nevus.

Surface Microscopy

Brown globules may be uniform in size, regular, and symmetrically distributed (benign pigmented lesions), or may be of different sizes and irregular spaced (dysplastic or malignant lesions). In the center or at the periphery of some lesions symmetric gray-blue globules can be found (Spitz nevi). In melanomas the globules are unevenly distributed. Reddish colored globules are highly suggestive of melanoma. A peripheral rim of globules is characteristic of enlarging nevi.

Histopathology

Nests of melanocytes/nevus cells with different levels of pigmentation are located at the dermoepidermal junction, the papillary, and the reticular dermis (Figs. 79, 80).

References

20; 24; 47; 82; 279; 314

Globules

Synonyms

Synonyms for globules are pigment globules, brown globules, multiple peripheral brown globules, and multiple blue-gray globules.

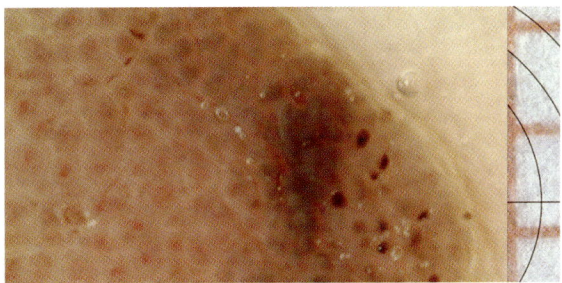

◘ **Fig. 79** Nodular melanoma (Clark level IV, Breslow thickness 1.48 mm) on the thigh shows irregular-shaped and distributed reddish to slate-gray globules throughout the lesion

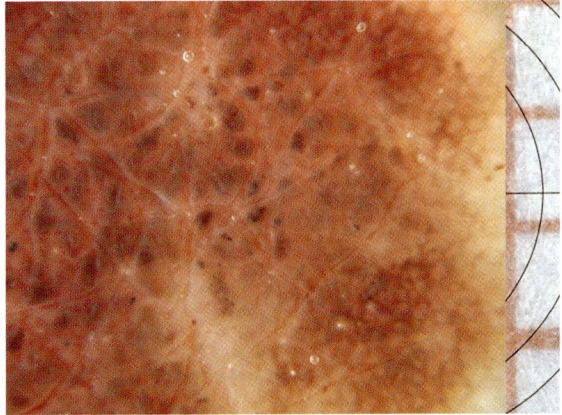

◘ **Fig. 80** A junctional nevus on the breast demonstrates multiple reddish brown to slate-gray globules

Definition

Globules are melanocytic lesions with round-to-oval, well-demarcated spherical shapes (usually >0.1 mm in diameter) that may be black, brown, or red.

Occurrence

Globules occur in benign as well as in dysplastic and malignant melanocytic lesions including Spitz nevus and recurrent nevus, but also in basal cell carcinoma (blue-gray to slate-gray ovoid pigment accumulations) and dermatofibroma (ring-like with a darker peripheral rim).

Surface Microscopy

In benign melanocytic lesions the globules (Figs. 81, 82) are regular in size and shape and quite evenly distrib-

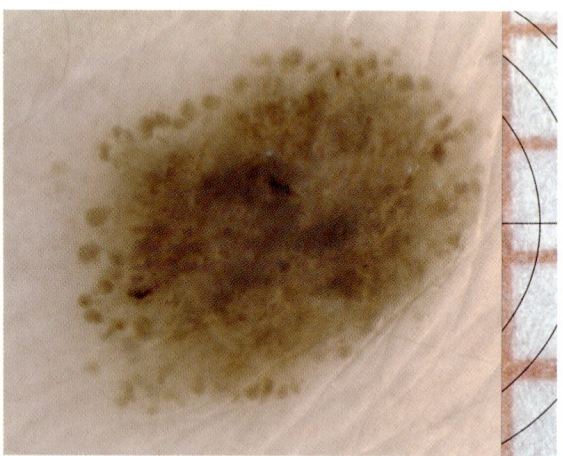

□ Fig. 81 Corona-like brown globules in Reed's nevus

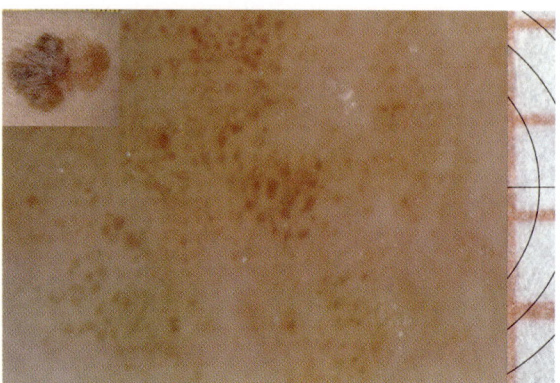

□ Fig. 82 Superficial spreading melanoma (Clark level II, Breslow thickness 0.4 mm) on the lower leg shows multiple irregularly pigmented and distributed brown globules

uted (frequently in the center of the lesion). Nests of pigmented cells within the dermal papillae are seen as brown globules in the mesh centers of the network. In melanomas they tend to vary in size, color, and shape, and they are irregularly distributed and frequently found in the periphery of lesions. A variant of dysplastic nevi shows multiple peripheral brown globules at the edge of the lesion. In Spitz nevi brown globules are often peripheral and multilayered. Well-defined multiple blue-gray globules occur in basal cell carcinoma with a specificity of about 97% (no pigment network is present). They may also be seen rarely in seborrheic keratoses. Ring-like globules with a darker peripheral rim can frequently be observed in dermatofibromas. The globule-like structures seen in dermatofibromas are due to the fact that the rete ridges are often flat, confluent, and hyperpigmented (post-inflammatory hyperpigmentation). The surrounding peripheral network is usually light-to-medium brown in color, fine and delicate, and gradually fades in the surrounding skin.

Histopathology

Histopathology shows nests of pigmented benign or atypical melanocytes, and clumps of melanin and/or melanophages situated in the lower epidermis, at the dermoepidermal junction, at the tips of the rete pegs, or in the papillary dermis. In basal cell carcinomas there are scattered and focal collections of melanin pigment within the tumor nests.

References

21; 137; 142; 143; 144; 183; 186; 188; 213; 218; 279; 280; 286; 298

Glomerular Vessels

Definition

Glomerular vessels form a glomerulus-like pattern of neovascularization within the papillary dermis.

Occurrence

Glomerular vessels occur as malignant melanoma, epidermotropic metastasis of malignant melanoma, basal cell carcinoma (Fig. 83), Bowen's disease, and squamous cell carcinoma (Fig. 84).

Surface Microscopy

The vascular density of the tumor is increased with dilated and elongated vessels during the process of neo-

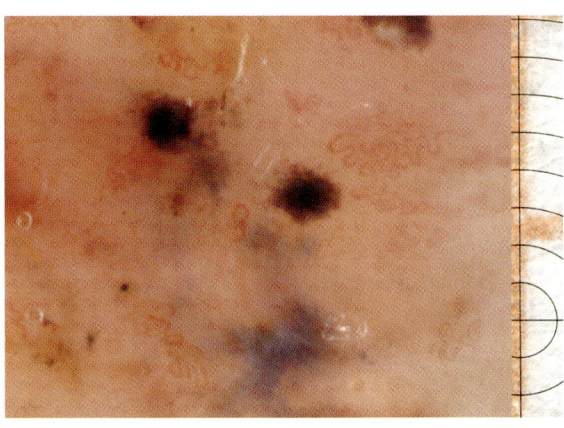

Fig. 83 Pigmented basal cell carcinoma on the lower leg shows glomerular vessels

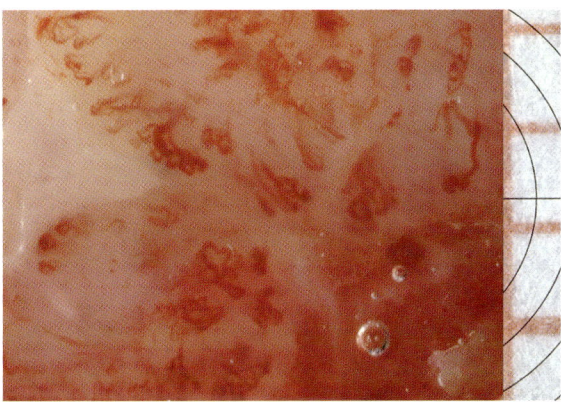

Fig. 84 Squamous cell carcinoma (pT2c, Broder's grade III) on the temple presenting with multiple glomerular vessels

vascularization, resulting in tortuous or glomerulus-like patterns of vessels.

Reference

160

Granular Layer

▶ Stratum granulosum.

Gray Streaks Surrounding the Lesion

Definition

Gray streaks surrounding the lesion consists of fine grayish streaks (melanoma cell necrosis) in the immediate surrounding tissues of a melanocytic lesion.

Surface Microscopy

There are fine grayish streaks (Fig. 85), up to 2 mm in length, that reflect through the epidermis in the periphery of the lesion. Short tree-like branchings of the streaks may be present.

Histopathology

Histopathology shows necrotic streaks of melanoma cells within lymphatic vessels and/or blood vessels in the dermis.

References

261; 262; 263

Gray-black and Blue-gray Ovoid Nests

Synonyms

Synonyms for gray-black and blue-gray ovoid nests are large blue-gray ovoid nests or slate-gray ovoid or larger areas.

Definition

Gray-black and blue-gray ovoid nests are well-circumscribed, confluent, or near-confluent pigmented ovoid or elongated areas, usually larger than globules (> 0.2 mm), more irregular in shape, and not closely connected to a pigmented tumor body.

Occurrence

Gray-black and blue-gray ovoid nests occur as pigmented basal cell carcinoma (> 50%; absence of a pigment network, typical vascular pattern; Figs. 86, 87), malignant melanoma (3%), and benign pigmented lesions (1%).

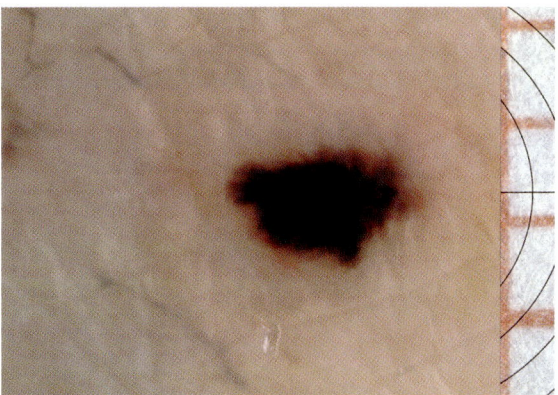

Fig. 85 In-transit melanoma metastasis on the thigh shows fine gray streaks surrounding the lesion

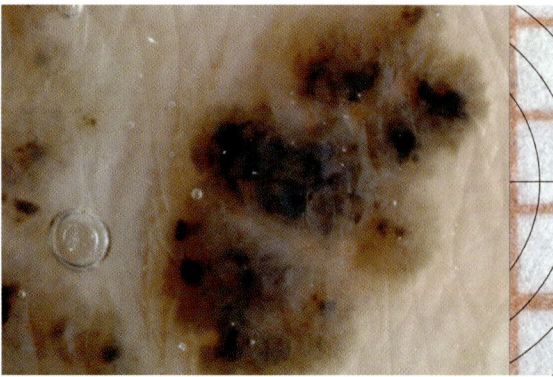

◘ **Fig. 86** This pigmented basal cell carcinoma on the trunk lacks a pigment network and shows gray-black or blue-gray ovoid nests and areas of leaf-like pigmentation

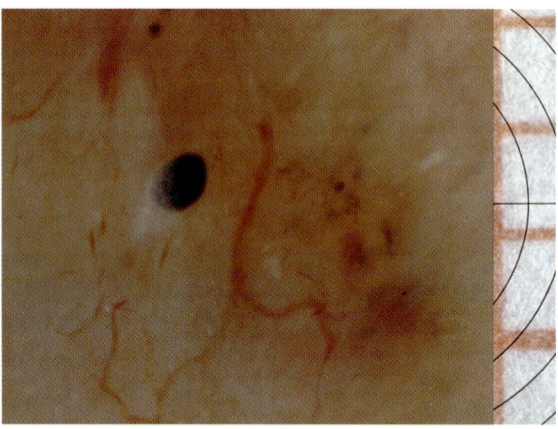

◘ **Fig. 87** Pigmented basal cell carcinoma on the forehead shows a large blue-gray ovoid nest

Histopathology

Melanin pigment is concentrated within large nests of tumor cells.

References

188; 218; 246

Gray-black Perifollicular Pigmentation

▶ Perifollicular pigment changes.

Gray-blue Trabecular Melanophages

▶ Trabeculae of melanophages.

Gray-blue/black Papillary Globules

▶ Target globules.

Grayish Patches

Synonym

The synonym for grayish patches is multiple grayish patches

Definition

Grayish patches are defined as irregularly localized grayish patches, > 0.35 mm in diameter, at the periphery or near the border of a melanocytic lesion.

Occurrence

Grayish patches occur as malignant melanomas and malignant melanoma metastases.

Surface Microscopy

Surface microscopy shows usually multiple irregular unstructured aggregates of grayish dense-appearing pigment concentrations (pigment dust) at the border of the lesion (Fig. 88).

Histopathology

Histopathology shows melanin aggregates in the dermis.

References

11; 143; 259; 260; 261

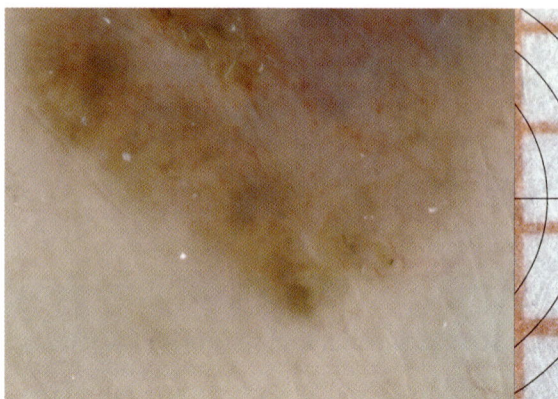

◘ **Fig. 88** Unclassified malignant melanoma on the upper arm (Clark level II, Breslow thickness 0.41 mm) shows irregular grayish patches near the border

Gyri

► Fissures and ridges.

Gyri and Sulci

► Fissures and ridges.

Hairpin-like-shaped Blood Vessels

Definition

These blood vessels are twisted and bended (or curved) vascular loops.

Occurrence

These vessels occur as keratoacanthoma (thick hairpins), seborrheic keratosis (fine hairpins in a cerebriform arrangement), molluscum contagiosum (linear or curvilinear vessels at the periphery), malignant melanoma (irregular hairpins), and hairpin-like loops in the nailfolds.

Surface Microscopy

In keratoacanthoma a corona of thick, twisted, and curved hairpin-like vessels can be seen (Fig. 89). Seborrheic keratoses often show a light halo surrounding the vessels. The white halo is mainly seen in keratinizing tumors and it is absent in melanocytic lesions that are supplied by vascular loops, i.e., amelanotic malignant melanoma and hypomelanotic Spitz nevus (in the center). Normal nailfold capillaries run parallel to the neighboring vessels, to the axis of the finger, and to the skin surface. The efferent side of the loop is slightly wider compared with the afferent side.

References

160; 311

Hairpin-like-shaped Corona

▶ Red corona.

Halo Nevus

Synonyms

Synonyms for Halo nevus are Sutton's nevus and leukoderma acquisitum centrifugum.

Definition

Halo nevus is a brown to reddish-brown melanocytic macule or dome-shaped papule with peripheral hypopigmentation.

Surface Microscopy

The brown pigmented oval macule or slightly raised papule is surrounded by a white corona (reduction or absence of melanocytes). Globules and dots are present in the center (Fig. 90).

Histopathology

There are nests of melanocytes at the dermoepidermal junction with or without a dermal component. The melanocytes may display slight nuclear atypia, espe-

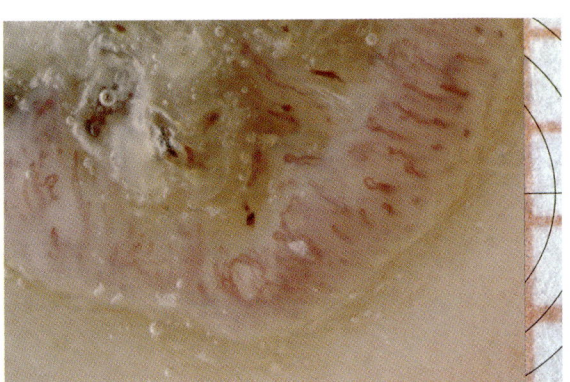

🔲 **Fig. 89** Keratoacanthoma on the upper arm shows a corona of hairpin-like-shaped blood vessels in the periphery of the lesion

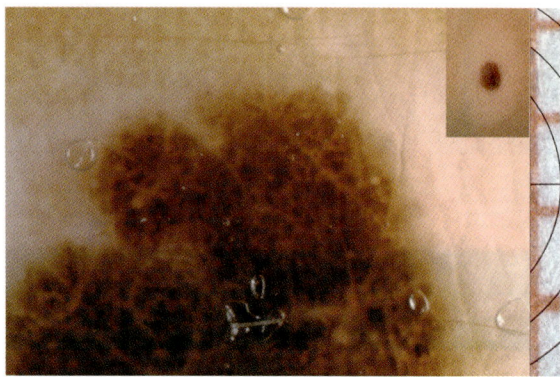

Fig. 90 Halo nevus of the compound type consists of multiple brown globules and blotches, and a peripheral hypopigmentation

cially those that are surrounded by lymphocytes. A dense symmetrically arranged and lichenoid lymphocytic infiltrate extends beneath the halo.

References

5; 118; 298

Hang-glider Sign

Definition

Dark triangular biting apparatus of Sarcoptes scabiei at the end of the subcorneal tunnel.

Reference

298

Hemangioma Senile

▶ Hemangiomas.

Hemangiomas

Synonyms

Synonyms for hemangioma are angioma, capillary hemangioma, and cavernous hemangioma.

Definition

Hemangiomas are benign tumors of blood vessels. Eruptive angiomas (senile hemangioma, cherry hemangioma, hemangioma senile, ruby spot) composed of capillary vessels are isolated or multiple, cherry-red to violaceous, flat or raised, sharply demarcated

lacunae (lagoons) and sometimes polyploidy papules (1–6 mm in diameter). Cavernous hemangiomas with large vascular spaces vary in size (1 cm to more than 10 cm) and may occur singly or multiply. They are already present at birth but can occur in later stages of life. Transitional forms can exist between vascular tumors and vascular nevi (i.e., hemangioma planum, nevus flammeus).

Surface Microscopy

The basic structure consist of multiple smooth-bordered red, purplish, blue-red (deeper in the dermis) or blue-black (thrombosed) blood sinuses (lacunes) which are homogeneous in color, without transepidermal melanin spreading, streaks, globules, or any trace of pigment network (Fig. 91). The dilated vascular spaces of the stratum papillare are separated by whitish-opaque fibrous septa. Partially or completely hemorrhagic dark blue to blue-black thrombotic plugs are common features within hemangiomas.

Histopathology

Convolution of capillaries (of the subpapillary plexus) or cavernous large vascular spaces lined with endothelium are seen within the upper dermis and/or subcutis. The tumors often contain mixed elements of capillary and cavernous sinuses.

References

136; 143

Hematolymphangioma

▶ Lymphangioma.

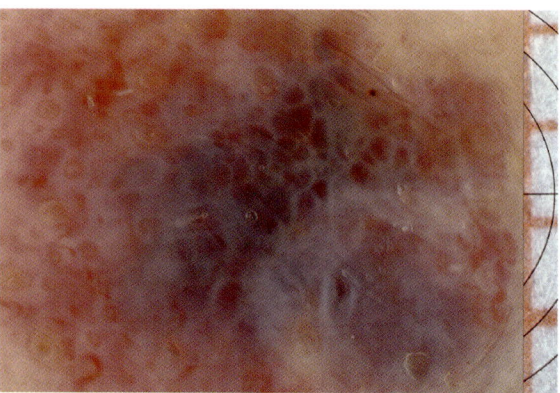

Fig. 91 Hemangioma capillare simplex on the cheek demonstrates multiple well-demarcated red to blue-red lacunae which are tightly clustered and partly separated by whitish-opaque septa. Note the multiple follicular plugs

Homogeneous Pattern

Definition

Homogeneous pattern is a diffuse homogeneous, brown, blue, gray-blue to gray-black, or reddish-black pigmentation of the lesion (partial or pigmentation throughout) without a pigment network or any other discernable structures.

Occurrence

Homogeneous pattern occurs as melanocytic nevi, blue nevi, combined nevi, Spitz nevi, Reed nevi, melanocytic nevi of the palms and soles, malignant melanoma (irregular), subungual benign and malignant melanocytic lesions (longitudinal pigmentation), as well as lentigo and drug-induced or ethnic nail pigmentation (grayish).

Surface Microscopy

A reddish periphery or a reddish homogeneous pattern can be a hint that the lesion is a Spitz nevus (zoned pattern), a malignant melanoma (zonal to irregular pattern), or a cutaneous metastasis of melanoma (Figs. 92, 93).

Histopathology

Homogeneous pattern shows homogeneous distribution of nested benign or malignant melanocytes, epithelioid, and/or spindle cells with different levels of pigmentation at the dermoepidermal junction and/or papillary dermis.

References

47; 82; 110; 139; 302

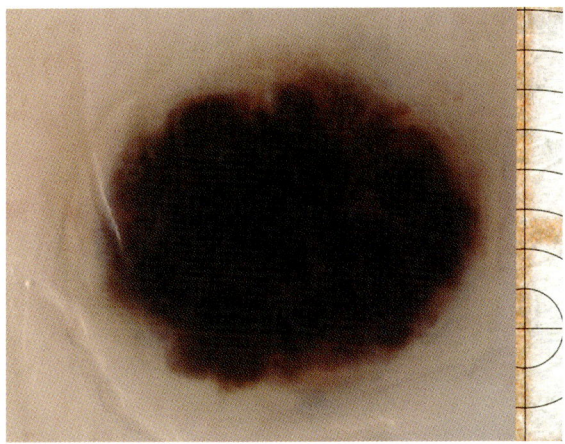

Fig. 93 A cutaneous metastasis of malignant melanoma with a reddish periphery and a central area of homogeneous gray-blue pigmentation

Homogeneous–Globular Pattern

Definition

Homogeneous–globular pattern is a melanocytic lesion that consists of a pigmented globular basic pattern that suggests benign alteration. Other typical features and criteria for melanocytic changes, e.g., pigment network and branched streaks, with the exception of dots and background pigmentation, are absent (Fig. 94).

Honeycomb-like Network

▶ Reticular pattern.

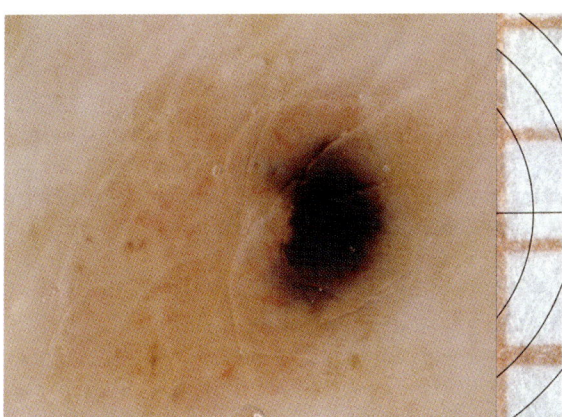

Fig. 92 Combined nevus with a focal area of homogeneous blue-gray pigmentation

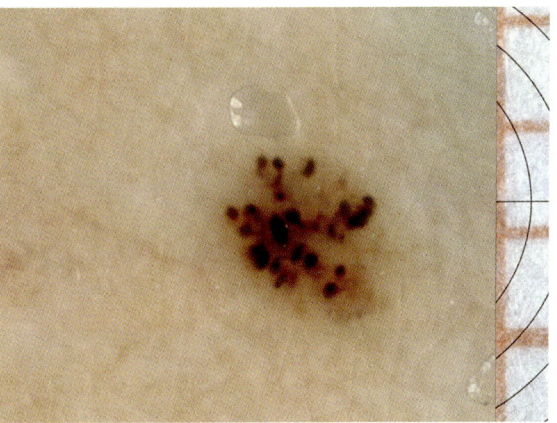

Fig. 94 Junctional nevus on the scapular region shows a homogeneous–globular pattern

Horny Layer

▶ Stratum corneum.

Hutchinson's Sign

Definition

Hutchinson's sign is the extension of subungual pigmentation to adjacent periungual skin in a case of melanonychia (micro-Hutchinson's sign: periungual pigmentation on the cuticle not evident with the naked eye).

Occurrence

Hutchinson's sign is acrolentiginous melanoma and is occasionally seen in benign nevi.

Surface Microscopy

Surface microscopy shows pigmentation of the cuticle in the area corresponding to the pigmented nail band (Fig. 95). That can be an irregular perionychial pigmentation (in advanced cases of malignant melanomas) or a pigmentation of the cuticle only (melanoma in situ).

References

141; 240; 302

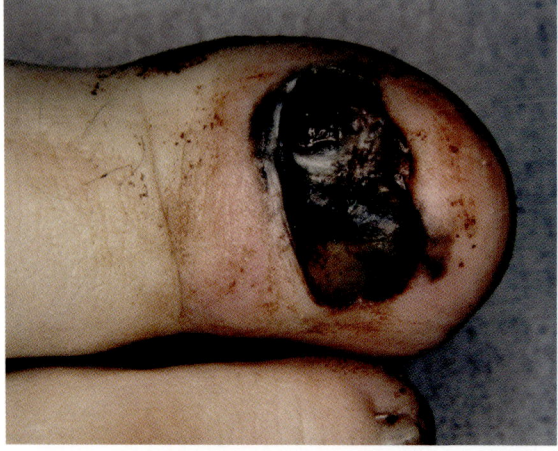

☐ **Fig. 95** Nail unit melanoma, ALM type, Clark's level III, 1.8 mm thickness in an adult's first toenail. Pigmentation of the cuticle and the periungual skin, typical of advanced melanoma (atypical Hutchinson's sign), is shown

Hypergranulosis

Hypergranulosis is increased thickness of the granular layer of the epidermis, usually associated with hyperkeratosis, foci of which occur in some diseases, e.g., lichen planus or verrucae vulgaris. In surface microscopy it creates a typical whitish-opaque hue.

Hyperkeratosis

Hyperkeratosis is an abnormal keratinization of the epidermis and mucous membranes resulting in thickening of the stratum corneum. Retention hyperkeratosis has a narrow stratum granulosum and a reduced desquamation of corneocytes, e.g., in ichthyosis. Proliferation hyperkeratosis with accelerated epidermopoiesis has thickened stratum corneum and usually an increased stratum granulosum, e.g., initial psoriatic plaques, advanced psoriasis (absence of the granular layer), and pityriasis rubra pilaris.

Hyperparakeratosis

Hyperparakeratosis is the normal keratinization of the epidermal horny layer in association with parakeratosis, i.e., qualitatively abnormal or incomplete keratinization of the corneocytes within the stratum corneum. Hyperparakeratosis may be observed in many scaling dermatoses such as psoriasis and subacute or chronic dermatitis. As to the epidermal transparency using surface microscopy, it depends upon the thickness of the horny layer.

Hyperpigmentation

Definition

Hyperpigmentation consists of circumscribed or diffuse brown, blue-gray (slate-gray), and black pigmented areas of the skin, within skin lesions or within interfollicular and perifollicular zones.

Occurrence

Hyperpigmentation occurs as Addison's disease (diffuse pigmentation in skin areas exposed to light), benign nevi (homogeneous), clinically atypical nevi (irregular), congenital melanocytic nevi (interfollicu-

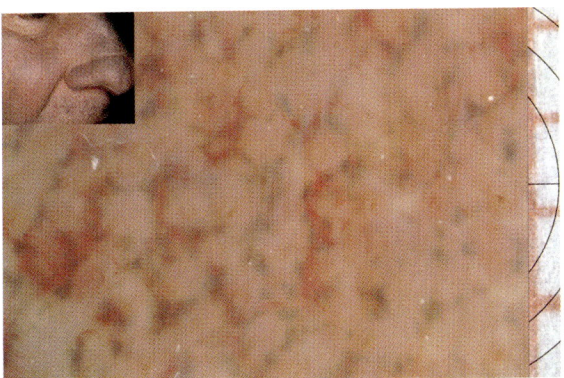

☐ **Fig. 96** Amiodaron-induced interfollicular and perivascular streaks or blotches of blue-gray to light-brown hyperpigmentation (lipofuscin) in facial skin

☐ **Fig. 97** Melanosis diffusa congenita on the forehead with follicles lying very close together shows interfollicular gray streaks, blotches, and annular–granular structures

lar, perifollicular), drug-induced hyperpigmentation (interfollicular and perivascular; Fig. 96), lentigo (homogeneous), malignant melanoma (irregular), melanodermitis (brownish-violet staining in areas exposed to the sun), melanosis (diffuse), melasma or chloasma (annular–granular pattern in facial regions; Fig. 97), phototoxic dermatitis (diffuse, lichenoid), postinflammatory pigmentation (diffuse), Spitz nevi (center, targetoid pattern), and Reed nevi (center, targetoid pattern).

References

47; 58; 174; 304

Hyperplastic Sebaceous Glands

▶ Crown vessels.

Hypogranulosis

Hypogranulosis is an abnormal thinning or vanishing of the epidermal stratum granulosum that normally consists of three cell layers, e.g., in psoriasis. The thickness of the stratum corneum also tends to be reduced.

In surface microscopy the epidermis becomes more translucent.

Hypokeratosis

An abnormal thinning of the stratum corneum of the epidermis, for instance in aging skin. Usually the thickness of the granular layer, normally consisting of three cell layers, tends also to be diminished. In surface microscopy the epidermis becomes more transparent, allowing a better inspection of the more deeply localized dermal structures.

Hypopigmentation

Definition

Decrease in pigment within a melanocytic lesion. The hypopigmented region has less pigmentation than the rest of the overall lesion pigmentation. In benign lesions this feature is regular and symmetrically located. In melanoma hypopigmentation has an irregular distribution.

Reference

82

Ink-spot Lentigo

▶ Solar lentigo.

In-vivo Histology

Synonym

The synonym for in-vivo histology is vital histology. The term "vital histology" was first used by Franz Ehring (1953), the originator of the modern videomicroscopy, in cooperation with Johannes Schumann (1965). Using an intravital stereomicroscope in combination with a high-resolution epiluminescence microscope illuminator (magnification up to about 1000×) and a TV-video system, it was possible to observe and interpret not only histological or cytological aspects in the skin but also the living conditions, e.g., the blood stream, and the function of the peri- and subcapillary tissue. A checklist with six in-vivo-histology criteria to diagnose malignancy of melanocytic lesions was established by Ehring et al. [92] (see Table 9).

References

88; 90; 91; 92; 264; 265

In-transit Melanoma Metastases

▶ Malignant melanoma metastases, cutaneous.

Inverse Network

▶ Negative network.

Table 9 In-vivo histology criteria of malignant melanoma. (Modified from [92])

In all layers of the epidermis, including the stratum corneum, there is melanin pigmentation
The borders of the dermal papillae are not demarcated from the surrounding tissues
Heavily pigmented cell nests which extend into the dermis
Increased and irregularly branched capillary network
Reddish to brownish hemorrhages
Inflammatory infiltrate

The appearance of at least two criteria are indicative of malignancy

Irregular Area of Slate-gray Target Globules

▶ Target globules.

Irregular Blotches

▶ Blotches.

Irregular Depigmentation

▶ Depigmentation.

Irregular Diffuse Pigmentation

▶ Diffuse pigmentation.

Irregular Dots

Definition

Irregular black/brown dots (< 0.1 mm in diameter) are variously sized and asymmetrically distributed within a melanocytic lesion.

Occurrence

In-transit melanoma metastases occurs as malignant melanoma (multiple irregular brown dots are a highly indicative feature for an invasive melanoma) and dysplastic nevi.

Surface Microscopy

Surface microscopy shows aggregations of well-defined irregularly distributed dark-brown dots (Fig. 98).

Histopathology

Histopathology shows suprabasal (intraepidermal) collections of pigment, mainly melanoma cells.

References

26; 188

Irregular Dots/Globules

▶ Dots; globules.

Irregular Extensions

▶ Pseudopods.

Irregular Linear–Polymorphous Vessels

▶ Irregular vessels.

Irregular Network

▶ Network irregularity.

Irregular Pattern, Nails

Definition

Subungual pattern of longitudinal brown-to-black lines with irregular thickness, spacing, discoloration, and disruption of the normal parallel pattern.

Occurrence

Irregular pattern in nails signifies nail-unit melanoma (prominent), occasionally in benign subungual nevi (indistinct).

Surface Microscopy

The superimposed lines on a brown background coloration are heterogeneous and asymmetrically distributed, varying in color, spacing, and thickness. In some areas the bands have a curved shape or abruptly interrupted pigmentation (Fig. 99).

Reference

302

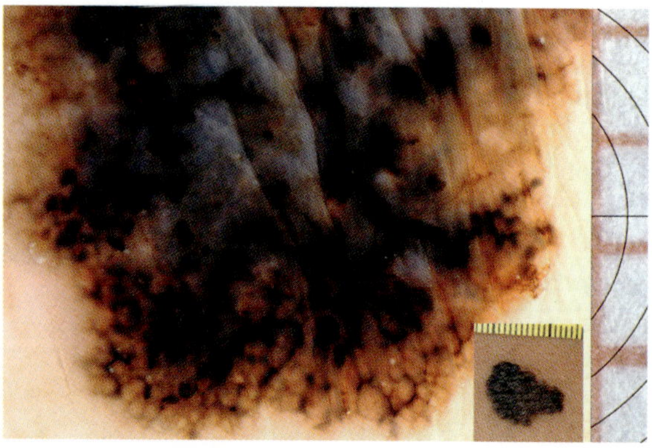

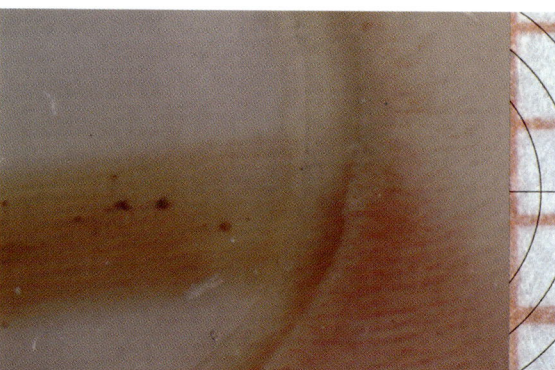

■ **Fig. 98** Unclassified malignant melanoma on the dorsum (Clark level II, Breslow thickness 0.39 mm) with irregularly distributed black dots varying in size, black branched streaks, and a black network with irregular holes and thick lines

■ **Fig. 99** Benign melanocytic nevus on the nail matrix with a brown color of the background and a regular parallel distribution of the overlying brown lines. The center of the bands are interrupted by brown (small nests of nevocytes) and slate-gray dots (blood spots)

Irregular Polymorphous Vessels

▶ Irregular vessels.

Irregular Streaks

▶ Radial streaming; pseudopods.

Irregular Vessels

Synonyms

Synonyms for irregular vessels are polymorphous vessels, irregular linear–polymorphous vessels, and linear irregular vessels.

Definition

Areas of small linear–irregular and/or polymorphous vessels running both parallel and vertical. They appear as red convoluted lines and small red dots simultaneously on a milky reddish background.

Occurrence

Irregular vessels occur as malignant melanoma (asymmetrically localized areas), amelanotic melanoma (the entire tumor is irregularly vascularized), cutaneous metastasis of malignant melanoma, Spitz nevus (the center of the lesion is irregular; Fig. 100), and Bowen's disease.

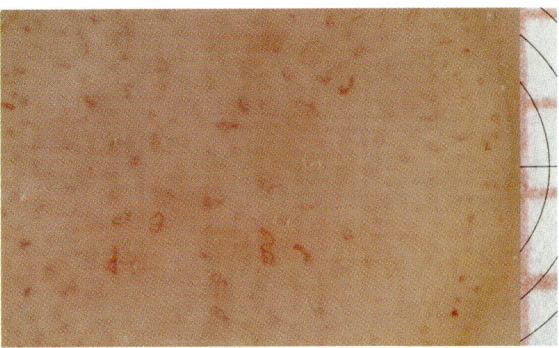

◘ **Fig. 100** Desmoplastic Spitz nevus shows irregular polymorphous vessels in the center of the lesion

Surface Microscopy

Surface microscopy shows linear and irregularly shaped, sized, and distributed red structures mostly similar to Greek minuscules. Focal areas or a wide distribution of multiple polymorphous capillaries (absent white halo surrounding the blood vessels) may be observed.

References

160; 191; 262; 298

Irritated Seborrheic Keratosis

▶ Seborrheic keratoses.

Jelly Sign

Synonym

The synonym for jelly sign is jelly-like border.

Definition

With a jelly sign the pigment appears to be on the skin surface, much like a jelly smear covering the skin (Fig. 101).

Occurrence

Jelly sign occurs as lentigo senilis, flat endophytic (adenoid–reticular) seborrheic keratoses.

Reference

298

Junctional Nevus

Definition

A junctional nevus is a sharply demarcated, flat, or slightly elevated round to oval macule, usually smaller than < 8 mm in diameter, and light to dark brown in color (Fig. 102). The histological examination demonstrates proliferation of three or more melanocytes in aggregation at the dermoepidermal junction.

Surface Microscopy

Surface microscopy shows symmetric reticular pattern that often fades at the periphery (faded regular edge). There may be areas of homogeneous pigmentation with regularly distributed dots (heavily pigmented keratinocytes) and globules (nests of melanocytes), usually in the center of the lesion.

◘ **Fig. 101** Jelly-like border (upper left side of the lesion) of an infraorbital lentigo senilis

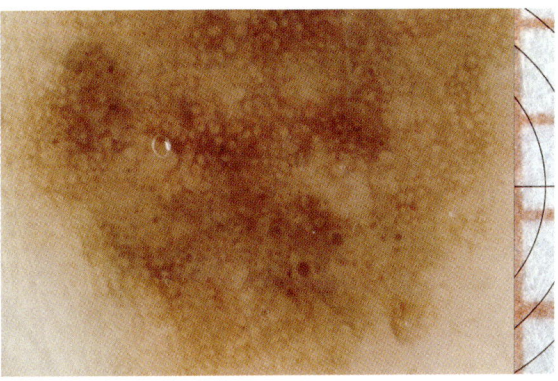

◘ **Fig. 102** Junctional nevus with a regular pigment network and regularly distributed brown globules (nests of nevocytes at the dermoepidermal junction)

Histopathology

Well-defined nests of melanocytes that in time descend into the dermis are localized at the dermoepidermal junction of elongated rete ridges. The keratinocytes may show increased melanin. Often melanophages are found in the upper dermis. Lamellar fibrosis and a mild lymphocytic infiltrate in the papillary dermis may be present.

References

38; 82; 118

Keratinocyte

Definition

Keratinocyte is the main constituent of the epidermis that produces keratin in the process of differentiating into the fully keratinized corneocyte of the stratum corneum (horny layer).

Keratosis Actinica

▸ Actinic keratosis.

Keratosis Follicularis

▸ Darier's disease.

Keratosis Senilis

▸ Actinic keratosis.

Keratosis Solaris

▸ Actinic keratosis.

Lacunae

Synonyms

Synonyms for lacunae are lacunes, red-blue areas, vascular lobules, blood sinuses, lagoon-like structures, and red lagoons.

Definition

Vascular lesions with multiple sharply demarcated ovoid blood sinuses of various sizes and colors (red to red-blue or red-black) that are clustered, partially grouped, or scattered throughout the lesion.

Occurrence

Lacunae occur as senile angiomas (cherry hemangiomas), hemangiomas, and angiokeratomas.

Surface Microscopy

The red to blue-red vascular lobules are separated by whitish-opaque septa (fibrous scar-like depigmentation surrounding the vascular spaces). Hemangiomas that had developed a partial thrombosis can acquire a focal blue-black or red-black color and resemble melanomas.

Histopathology

Histopathology shows increased and dilated vascular spaces (blood sinuses, lacunae; Fig. 103) in the stratum papillare.

References

136; 186; 261; 271

Lagoon-like Structures

► Lacunae.

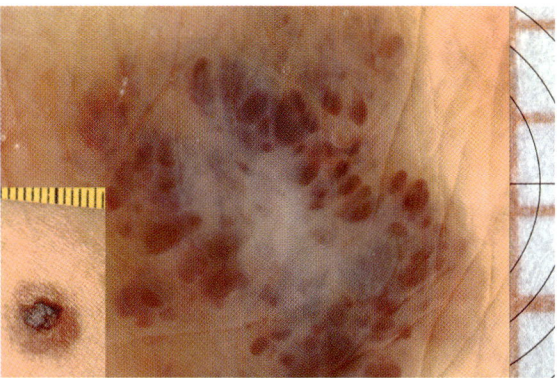

Fig. 103 Angiokeratoma in the scapular region consists of well-demarcated red to blue-red lacunae. The lesion has a central area of a whitish yellow hue suggestive of a coexistent hyperkeratosis

Lagoons

► Lacunae.

Large Blue-gray Ovoid Nests

► Gray-black and blue-gray ovoid nests.

Lattice-like Pattern

Definition

Lattice-like pattern consists of melanocytic lesions of the palms and soles with parallel pigmented lines along the furrows that are bridged by crossing the ridges. It is a variant of the parallel furrow pattern.

Occurrence

Lattice-like pattern occurs as mainly benign melanocytic nevi on volar and plantar skin.

Surface Microscopy

Surface microscopy shows a linear pattern with parallel lines along the furrows in combination with brownish dotted or linear pigmentation crossing the ridges (Fig. 104).

Histopathology

Nests of nevus cells are aggregated around the crista profunda limitans that lies below the surface furrows. In addition, there are pigmented cells within the crista superficialis (ridge).

References

56; 110; 240

Leaf-like Areas

Synonyms

Synonyms for leaf-like areas are maple-leaf-like areas, maple-leaf areas, and maple-leaf-like structures.

Definition

Leaf-like areas are pigmented lesions with brown to gray-blue discrete bulbous blobs or extensions connected at a base area, forming a maple-leaf-like pattern.

Occurrence

Leaf-like areas occur as pigmented basal cell carcinoma.

Surface Microscopy

The distribution of the gray-brown to gray-blue (slate gray) discrete pigmented leaf-like pattern reminds one of the shape of fingers or finger pads (Fig. 105). Sometimes the bulbous extensions of the leaf-like structures look like pseudopods, but in contrast to melanocytic lesions, a pigment network is absent and they usually do not arise from a confluent pigmented tumor.

Histopathology

Histopathology shows nests of discrete pigmented epithelial nodules of basal cell carcinoma (Fig. 106).

References

15; 21; 31; 55; 142; 143; 154; 183; 186; 187; 200; 211; 213; 218; 280; 281; 282; 285; 298; 315

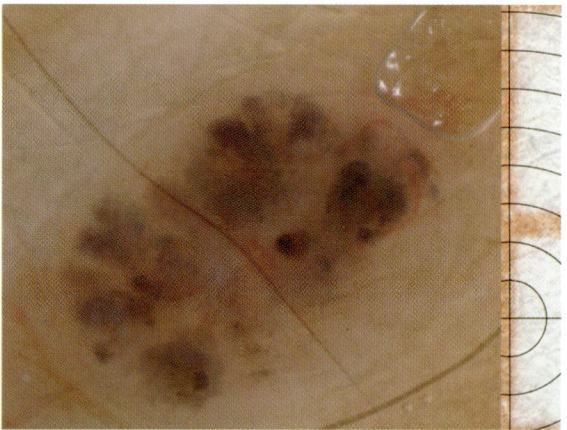

Fig. 105 Pigmented basal cell carcinoma in the scapular region shows a slate-gray leaf-like pattern

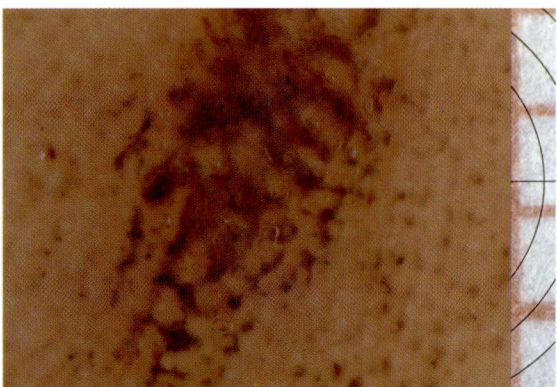

Fig. 104 Junctional nevus shows a lattice-like pattern

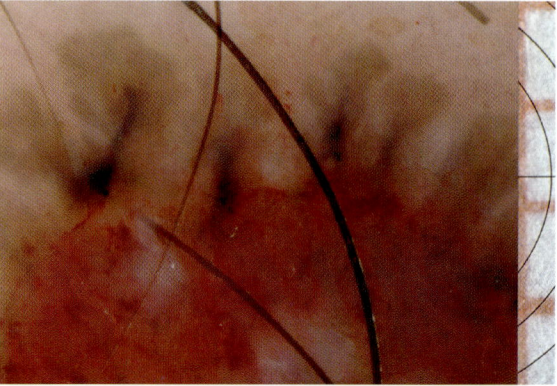

Fig. 106 Pigmented basal cell carcinoma on the thorax shows two colors of maple leaf-like areas, light brown and slate gray

Lentigo Maligna and Lentigo Maligna Melanoma

Synonyms

Synonyms for lentigo maligna and lentigo maligna melanoma are melanotic freckle, Hutchinson's freckle, and Dubreuilh tumor.

Definition

Lentigo maligna is a macular in-situ melanoma that results from proliferating neoplastic melanocytes within the epidermis of sun-exposed skin. Lentigo maligna melanoma comprises a background of lentigo maligna on which a confluence of melanocytes develops at the dermoepidermal junction and extends into the dermis.

Surface Microscopy

Surface microscopy shows features favoring lentigo maligna and lentigo maligna melanoma are as follows: hyperpigmented slate-gray to black rims surrounding the follicular openings in an asymmetric fashion (representing an uneven descent of atypical melanocytes). In addition, there may be individual grayish-black coloration of the central follicular plugs, interfollicular gray to blue-gray annular–granular pattern (dark rhomboidal structures and streaks, caused mainly by melanin in macrophages; Fig. 107), slate-gray dots and globules, white scar-like areas (regression pattern), and milky red areas indicating tumor progression (in advanced tumors), increased obliteration, and destruction of the pilosebaceous apparatus.

Histopathology

Histopathology of lentigo maligna shows that the actinically damaged epidermis is atrophic and occurs on a background of dermal solar elastosis. There is a proliferation of atypical melanocytes at the basal layer, with extension higher in the epidermis and in the adnexal structures. The basement membrane is intact. The dermis shows actinic damage with elastosis, melanophages, pigment incontinence, and a lymphocytic infiltrate. Lentigo maligna melanoma is similar to lentigo maligna but with obvious invasion into the dermis.

References

118; 128; 271

Lentigo Senilis

▶ Solar lentigo.

Lentigo Simplex

Definition

Lentigo simplex is a sharply demarcated small flat and round-to-oval area of reticular hyperpigmentation usually less than 5 mm in diameter.

Surface Microscopy

Surface microscopy shows strongly pigmented regular and symmetrical network pattern with thickened webs and often dilated holes in some parts. Areas of gray-blue pigmentation (melanophages), regular dots, and sometimes globules are observed at the center (Fig. 108).

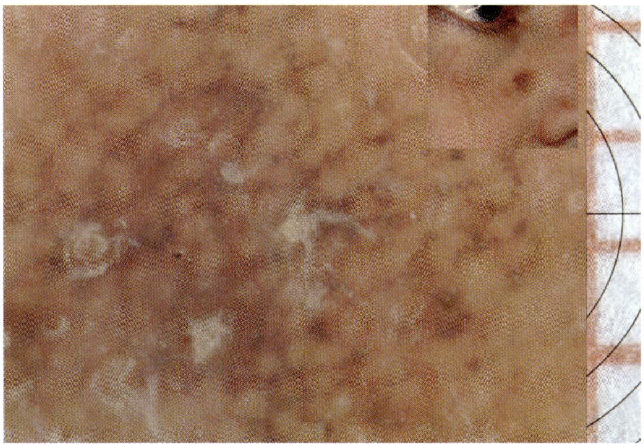

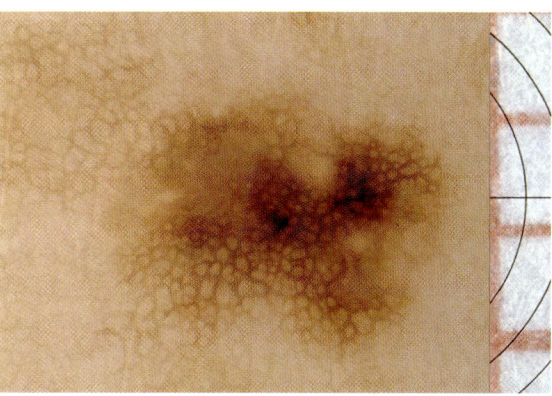

◘ **Fig. 107** Lentigo maligna melanoma on the infraorbital region (Clark level II, Breslow thickness 0.2 mm) represents an annular–granular pattern, slate-gray dots, and keratinized follicular openings

◘ **Fig. 108** Lentigo simplex, localized on sun-pigmented skin of the regio infrascapularis, shows a regular network pattern with a black dot in the center of the lesion

Histopathology

Histopathology shows elongation of the rete ridges with an increased number of basal layer melanocytes producing increased melanin. There is a mild fibroplasia and incontinence of pigment in the papillary dermis.

References

82; 118

Lesion Surrounded by Gray Streaks

▶ Gray streaks surrounding the lesion.

Leukoderma Acquisitum Centrifugum

▶ Halo nevus.

Lichen Planus

Synonym

The synonym for lichen planus is lichen ruber planus.

Definition

Lichen planus is a subacute or chronically progressive, inflammatory-red, polygonal papular skin eruption with a circumscribed thickening of the keratohyalin-containing cell layer of the stratum granulosum (hypergranulosis).

Surface Microscopy

On surface microscopy milky-white opaque Wickham striae are rounded, arboriform, reticular, or annular, sometimes obscuring the underlying structures (Figs. 109, 110). Projections of the border may be comb-like or ramified, and they are surrounded by radially arranged capillaries. Advanced lesions may show multiple blue-gray or brown dots (dermal melanophages) overlying hypopigmented areas.

Histopathology

Histopathology shows that the stratum corneum of the acanthotic epidermis is orthokeratotic associated with a thickened stratum granulosum (hypergranulosis). The epidermis often shows individual dyskeratotic cells. There is hydropic degeneration of the basal keratinocytes. Melanin is released from the degenerated basal cells and is engulfed by macrophages (melano-

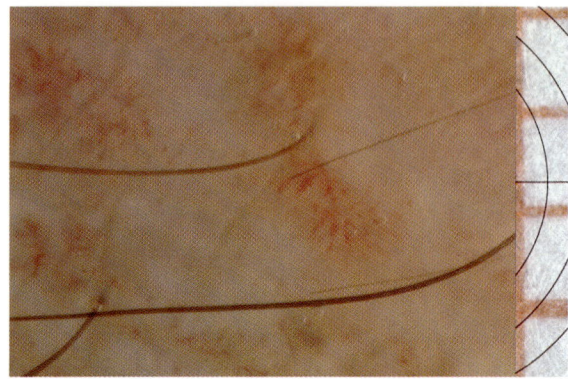

■ **Fig. 109** Lichen planus on the forearm shows reticular whitish-opaque areas surrounded by radial capillaries

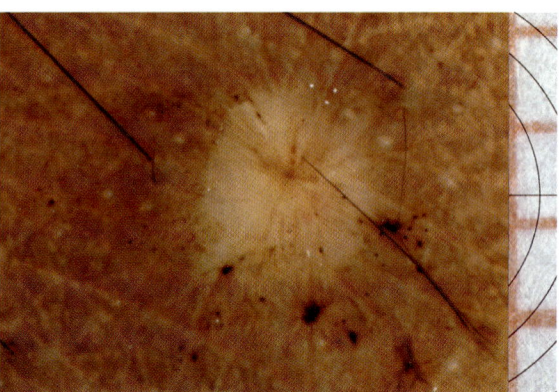

■ **Fig. 110** Advanced lichen planus on the forearm of a black woman represents a whitish-opaque center surrounded by brown dots

phages) in the dermis. A band-like inflammatory infiltrate beneath the epidermis is typical.

References

27; 306; 307; 308; 311

Lichen Planus-like Keratosis

▶ Seborrheic keratoses.

Lichenoid Actinic Keratosis

▶ Actinic keratosis.

Linear–Irregular Vessels

▶ Irregular vessels.

Liver Spot

▶ Solar lentigo.

Lupus Erythematosus

▶ Autoimmunogenic keratinocytolysis.
▶ Nailfold capillaries, alterations.

Lupus Erythematosus Chronicus Discoides

▶ Autoimmunogenic keratinocytolysis.
▶ Tack phenomenon.

Lymphangioma

Synonym
The synonym for lymphangioma is hematolymph-angioma.

Definition
Lymphangioma is a malformation of lymphatic vessels with translucent cavities or cyst-like shapes (pseudovesicles) varying in size within a circumscribed region.

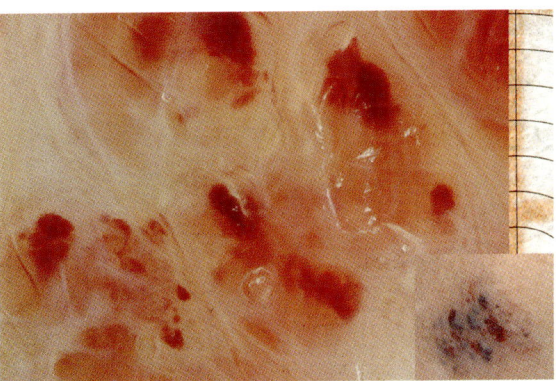

▣ **Fig. 111** A lymphangioma on the scapular region shows sharply demarcated yellowish to red lacunae

Surface Microscopy
Surface microscopy shows simultaneous presence of yellowish to skin-colored (lymph) and red (blood) sharply demarcated lacunae (lagoons, sinuses, lakes; Fig. 111).

Histopathology
Histopathology shows a combination of cavernous dilated and closely packed lymph vessels lined with endothelial cells and larger vascular channels which are in the various layers of the skin.

References
262; 298

Malignant Melanoma

Definition

Malignant melanoma consists of malignant, macularly elevated papules, and nodular or rarely depressed melanocytic lesions with variable colors. The atypical intraepidermal melanocytes may spread horizontally in the epidermis (pagetoid spread) or vertically into the dermis, or in both dimensions.

Surface Microscopy

Instead of being relatively uniformly brown, like melanocytic lesions, melanomas are variegated in brown colors and other colors such as black, blue, and pink. Usually a multicomponent pattern of three or more distinctive features can be seen (Fig. 112). Atypical pigment network, irregular dots and globules, irregular streaks (pseudopods, radial streaming), irregular blotches, regression structures, blue-white veil, and atypical vascular architecture are common in invasive melanomas (ABCD-E scoring system, ABCD rule, ABC point list of dermoscopy, enhanced ABCD-E scoring system, malignant melanoma and dysplastic nevi–ELM scoring system, Menzies' method, seven-point checklist, three-point checklist).

Histopathology

Malignant melanoma is characterized by individual normal or atypical melanocytes and nests of melanocytes that are not equidistant from one another, vary markedly in size and shape, tend to confluence, and fail to mature with progressive descent into the dermis. Atypical melanocytes are found at all levels of the epidermis and they are also located within the folliculosebaceous units and eccrine ducts. In the papillary dermis there may be some fibroplasias as well as a lymphocytic infiltrate of melanophages. The neoplastic melanocytes may descend from the epidermis into the dermis.

References

4; 5; 9; 28; 40; 58; 67; 69; 78; 80; 82; 85; 97; 98; 107; 113; 118; 153; 163; 181; 199; 204; 209; 212; 225; 227; 233; 266; 277; 292; 294; 313; 320; 322

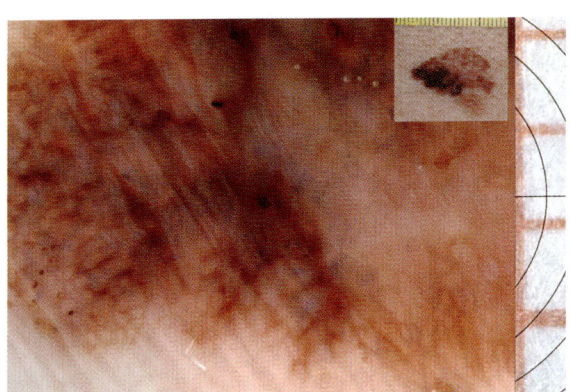

◩ **Fig. 112** Malignant melanoma (SSM, Clark level II, Breslow thickness 0.27 mm) shows a multicomponent pattern with atypical pigment network, irregular dots and globules, regression structures (peppering), and a blue-gray veil

Malignant Melanoma and Dysplastic Nevi, ELM Scoring System

Definition

A system for differentiating malignant melanomas from dysplastic nevi by assigning a point value to the findings on surface microscopic examination of the lesions (Table 10).

References

13; 255; 257; 258; 262

Table 10 Epiluminescent microscopic scoring system for melanomas and dysplastic nevi

Characteristic	Point value
Multiple grayish patches (> 0.35 mm)	11
Saccular pattern (red-blue, reddish-brownish, blue-gray)	11
Blue-white veil	10
Pseudotrabeculae of blue-gray granules (melanophages)	10
Blue-gray or slate-gray reticular remnants	10
Microscopic ovoid blood lakes	8
Irregular area of slate-gray target globules	7
Plaster-of-Paris-like lacunae	7
Degenerative changes with blue-gray granules in the marginal area	7
Polymorphic angiectatic base pattern	7
Whitish or bluish opaque pattern	5
Blue-in-pink area	5
Area of polymorphic ectatic vessels	5
Pseudopod-like structures of the margin	5
Radial streaming (digitiform extrusions)	5
Brown/black dot on a blue background	5
Abrupt cut-off of the trabeculae	3
Dendritic grayish-blue trabeculae (melanophages)	3
Gray-blue shading in pink	3
Multicomponent pattern (> 2)	3

Points 6–10 = suspicious of dysplasia (in some cases may be melanoma); >10 = suggests malignant melanoma

Malignant Melanoma, Cutaneous Metastases

Definition

Cutaneous malignant melanoma metastases usually occur initially via the dermal lymphatics. A microscopic nidus of melanoma cells is separated from the primary tumor, enters the tissue spaces, and invades an afferent lymph channel or the surrounding skin. The malignant cells can penetrate the lymph vessels with less resistance than the thicker venules. The most proximal type of metastasis occurs in the dermal and subdermal lymphatic and vascular channels. More superficial melanomas, less than 1.5 mm in Breslow's thickness, have a lesser probability of developing cutaneous metastases. When the melanoma has spread from the primary site for a distance of 2–10 cm, the metastases are found in the regional drainage area (satellitosis; Fig. 113). An in-transit type of spread of the tumor occurs between the primary malignant lesion and the regional lymph nodes.

Surface Microscopy

The initial cutaneous malignant melanoma metastases are small, discrete, usually uncoalesced, rounded areas of pigmented or hypomelanotic and non-pigmented (amelanotic) papules measuring 1–3 mm in size. There may be only one (solitary metastasis; Fig. 114), a few, or as many as ten and more. At this stage a distinction between benign and malignant melanocytic lesions is often difficult or impossible to make. A transepidermal elimination of melanin may obscure the underlying structures. Highly specific surface microscopic features of cutaneous metastases (malignant melanoma metastases, surface microscopy features) are as follows: saccular pattern (red-blue, red-light brown, reddish-brownish-gray, blue-gray, dark brown to black); red-brown globules irregular in size and color (indicating vascularized tumor cell nests); polymorphic angiec-

Fig. 113 Satellite metastasis of a malignant melanoma on the scapular region mimicks a blue nevus

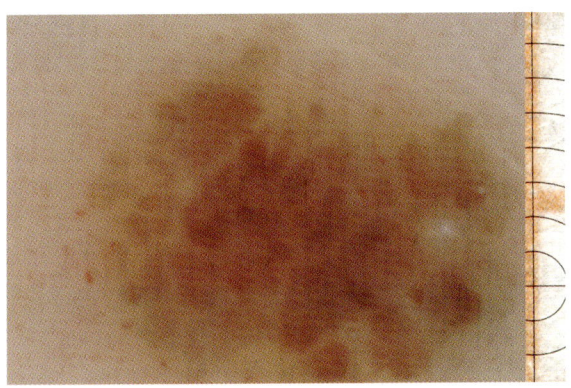

Fig. 114 Solitary cutaneous melanoma in-transit metastasis on the forearm shows a brownish saccular pattern and a red-dotted corona

tatic base pattern (Fig. 115) and/or aneurysms; areas of polymorphic ectatic vessels running parallel to the skin surface; peripheral erythema (red corona); microscopic ovoid blood lakes; gray streaks surrounding the lesion (melanoma cell infarcts); grayish patches; and homogeneous pattern (brown or blue to black).

Histopathology

The initial tumors are often solitary lesions localized in the stratum papillare and are not connected with the overlying epidermis. The adjacent epidermis may show collarette formation. In more advanced lesions the tumor may show epidermotropism with pagetoid features indistinguishable from primary melanomas. Tumor vascularity is often greater at the border than in the center.

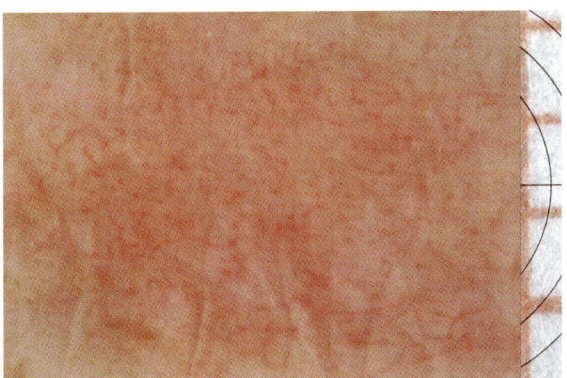

Fig. 115 Melanoma in-transit metastasis on the forearm shows a polymorphic angiectatic base pattern on a light-brown background

References

1; 4; 11; 16; 30; 31; 42; 74; 102; 125; 134; 143; 151; 154; 156; 158; 162; 182; 184; 186; 208; 211; 228; 234; 251; 252; 255; 257; 259; 260; 261; 287; 296; 298; 300; 317; 323

Malignant Melanoma Metastases: Surface Microscopy Features

Early cutaneous malignant melanoma metastases are small, discrete, usually uncoalesced, rounded areas of pigmented or hypomelanotic and non-pigmented (amelanotic) metastases measuring 1–3 mm in size. There may be only one (solitary metastasis), a few, or as many as ten and more. Often the distinction between benign and malignant melanocytic lesions is difficult or impossible to make. To facilitate the diagnosis specific surface microscopic variables are considered (Table 11).

References

4; 16; 125; 134; 151; 263

Table 11 Surface microscopy variables of cutaneous melanoma metastases

Feature	Specificity (%)	Sensitivity (%)
Saccular pattern (red-blue, red-light-brown, reddish-brownish-gray, blue-gray, dark brown to black)	96.0	40.0
Basic pattern of polymorphic vessels and/or aneurysms of the vessels	98.0	43.3
Areas of polymorphic and/or ectatic vessels running parallel to skin surface	92.0	40.0
Peripheral erythema	96.0	46.4
Microscopic ovoid blood lakes	100.0	10.0
Lesion surrounded by gray streaks (melanoma/cell infarcts)	100.0	20.0
Peripherally localized grayish patches	100.0	20.0

Homogeneous bluish pattern not evaluated

Malpighian Rete

► Rete ridges.

Maple-leaf-like Areas

► Leaf-like areas.

Maple-leaf-like Structures

► Leaf-like areas.

Marks Sign

Definition

Marks sign is dermatitis herpetiformis (Duhring) on acral sites showing multiple bizarre red brown spots (tiny punctate hemorrhages), usually along the lateral and medial aspects of the palm or sole.

References

133; 177; 236

Melanin

Definition

The melanin-producing melanocytes are located in the basal layer of the epidermis. The brownish pigment (eumelanin and pheomelanin) made in melanosomes is transferred to keratinocytes resulting in pigmentation of the epidermis.

Surface Microscopy

The color of the melanin depends upon its histological depth within the skin and the density of the pigment. Melanin appears black when located in the stratum corneum, dark brown within the epidermis, tan at or near the dermoepidermal junction, gray within the papillary dermis, and blue when it is located in the mid- to lower dermis.

References

44; 118

Melanin Pigmentation

► Melanin.

Melanocytes

A melanin-pigment-producing cell derives from the neuroectoderm, interspersed between the basal cells along the basement membrane of the epidermis. The cell possesses dendritic branching processes (dendrites) by which the melanosomes are transferred to the neighboring keratinocytes, resulting in the pigmentation of the skin.

Melanocytic Algorithm for Differentiating in Pigmented Lesions

Definition

This is a flow chart for stepwise melanocytic algorithm for differentiation between melanocytic and non-melanocytic lesions (see Table 12). In the first step it

◘ Table 12 Dermatoscopic algorithm—melanocytic vs non-melanocytic lesions. (Adapted from [298])	
Pigment network	Melanocytic skin lesions
Branched streaks	
Aggregated globules (exception: dermatofibroma and supernumerary nipple)	
Steel blue areas	Blue nevus
Pseudohorncysts	Seborrheic keratosis
Pseudofollicular openings	Gyri and sulci
Fingerprint-like pattern	
Moth-eaten border	
Jelly-like border	
Red, blue-red, or red-black lagoons	Hemangioma (often thrombosed)
Maple-leaf-like structures	Basal cell carcinoma
Larger arborizing or fine superficial vessels	
Slate gray ovoid structures or larger areas	
Spoke-wheel pattern	
Ulceration	
Melanocytic skin lesion	

is important to determine whether the three structural components – pigment network, pigmented aggregated globules, and branched streaks – are present. When the three structures are absent, one searches for the other criteria. At point 6 the pigmented lesions that cannot be positively identified remain. In most cases these components are of melanocytic origin and must be evaluated with regard to their malignant potential.

References

154; 280; 298

Melanoma Cell Infarct

▶ Gray streaks surrounding the lesion.

Melanocytic Nevus with Irregular Architecture

▶ Dysplastic nevus.

Melanodermitis

▶ Hyperpigmentation.

Melanoma in Association with Melanocytic Nevus

Definition

This is malignant melanoma that develops in association with a pre-existing melanocytic nevus.

Surface Microscopy

There are benign (e.g., pigment network, branched streaks, globules, dots) and malignant parts of melanocytic features. Mainly saccular pattern, milky-red globules (Fig. 116) or areas (neovascularization of malignant cell nests), white regression patterns, asymmetric darker zones, and an abrupt cut-off of the pigment network at the periphery suggest malignancy.

References

290; 298

Melanoma with Marked Regression

Synonym

The synonym for melanoma with marked regression is regressing malignant melanoma.

Definition

Melanoma with marked regression is malignant melanoma with extensive regressive changes that lead to a predominantly amelanotic lesion.

Surface Microscopy

Peppering zones that consist of multiple blue-gray to slate-gray aggregated dots or granules (melanophages) together with scar-like regression patterns and irregular vessels can be observed (Fig. 117). Globules, branched streaks, and peripheral pigment network structures may be absent.

References

262; 298

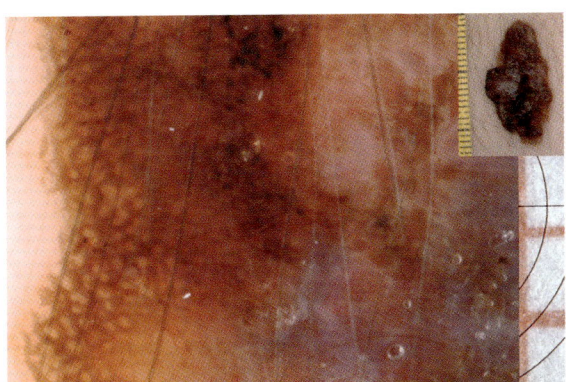

◘ **Fig. 116** Superficial spreading melanoma (Clark level IV, Breslow thickness 3.6 mm) in association with a papillomatous nevus on the trunk shows an abrupt cut-off of the network, milky-red globules, and a reddish-brown saccular pattern

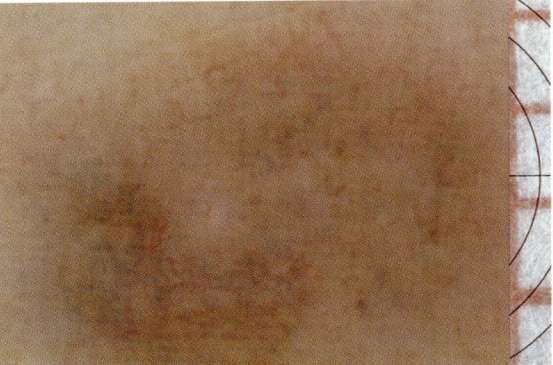

◘ **Fig. 117** Regressive superficial spreading melanoma on the calf of the leg (Clark level IV, Breslow thickness 0.44 mm) multiple slate-gray aggregated granules (melanophages), and irregular linear vessels on a light-brown background

Melanophage

Melanophage is a histiocyte of the dermis that has phagocytized melanin. On surface microscopy there is no transepidermal elimination of pigment, because melanophages do not release their incorporated melanin.

Melanosis

▶ Hyperpigmentation.

Melanosis Neviformis

Synonyms
Synonyms for melanosis neviformis are Becker's nevus and pigmented hairy epidermal nevus.

Definition
Melanosis neviformis is a unilateral gradually enlarging map-like melanocytic lesion also considered as a hamartoma with hypertrichosis, and smooth muscle components. The lesion contains melanin, but without associated nests of nevus cells. Melanophages in the upper dermis indicate pigment incontinence.

Reference
5

Melanosomes

Melanosomes are special cytoplasmatic organelles that form oval pigment granules ($0.2 \times 0.6\,\mu m$) within melanocytes, where the synthesis and later the storage of melanin occurs.

Melasma

▶ Hyperpigmentation.

Menzies' Method

Definition
Menzies' method is a simplified dermoscopy method for the diagnosis of melanoma (Table 13). This method gives a sensitivity of 92% and a specificity of 71% for

▣ Table 13 The Menzies method. (Modified from [189])
Negative features (in melanoma, neither can be found)
Symmetry of pigmentation pattern
Presence of only a single color
Positive features (at least one feature found)
Blue-white veil
Multiple brown dots
Pseudopods
Radial streaming
Scar-like depigmentation
Peripheral black dots/globules
Multiple (five to six) colors
Multiple blue-gray dots: "peppering"
Broadened network

the diagnosis of melanoma (containing both in-situ and invasive lesions).

References
24; 185; 188; 189

Menzies' Sign

▶ Moth-eaten border.

Metastatic Malignant Melanoma

▶ Malignant melanoma metastases, cutaneous.

Micro-Hutchinson's Sign

▶ Hutchinson's sign.

Microscopic Longitudinal Grooves, Nails

Definition
This consists of superficial microscopic fractures of the nail plate. The thin longitudinal whitish-opaque

fissures can be observed in several nail conditions (e.g., psoriasis; Fig. 118). They are not always super-imposed on a pigmented band and not indicative of any diagnosis.

Reference

302

Microscopic Ovoid Blood Lakes

▶ Ovoid blood lakes.

Miescher's Nevus

Definition

Dome-shaped, firm, nearly skin-colored compound or intradermal melanocytic nevus. It has a predominantly endophytic and wedge-shaped growth pattern. The nests, cords, and strands of melanocytes extend from beneath a thinned papillary dermis into the reticular dermis. Within the wedge, folliculosebaceous structures are spared by the melanocytes (Fig. 119). Under surface microscopy they are largely similar to poorly pigmented dermal nevi.

Reference

5

Milia-like Cysts

▶ Pseudohorncysts.

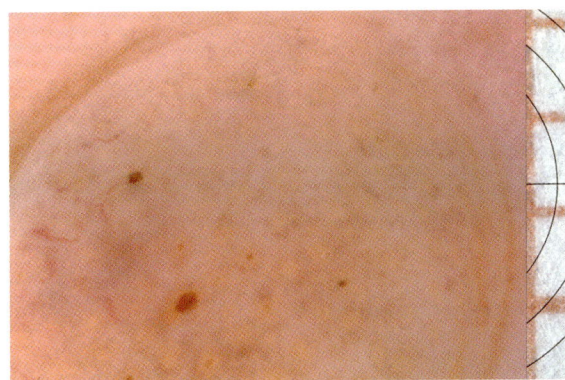

□ Fig. 119 Miescher's nevus on the nasolabial region represents yellowish to light-brown round structures (partly atrophic folliculosebaceous units), diffuse grayish-brownish pigmentation, and some ectatic vessels near the border

Milky-red Areas

Synonym

The synonym for milky-red areas is milky-red globules.

Definition

Milky-red areas are ill-defined or fuzzy milky-red areas or globules usually corresponding to well-vascularized tumor nests (tumor nodules) within an elevated part of a melanocytic lesion (Fig. 120).

Occurrence

Milky-red areas occur as malignant melanoma, Clark's nevus, and Spitz nevus.

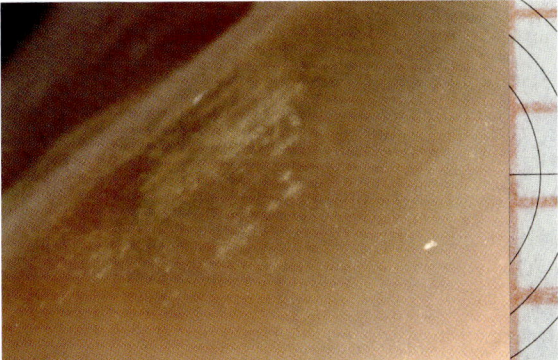

□ Fig. 118 Psoriasis of the nail plate shows longitudinal whitish-opaque fractures on a yellowish-brown coloration of the background (psoriatic oil spot)

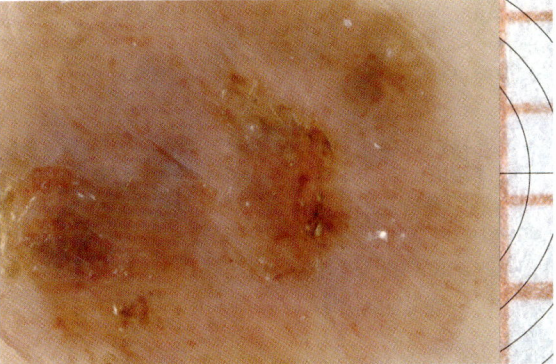

□ Fig. 120 Unclassified malignant melanoma (Clark level II, Breslow thickness 0.41 mm) on the upper arm shows blurred milky-red (well-vascularized) areas

References

143; 154; 160; 298

Milky-red Globules

▶ Milky-red areas.

Molluscum Contagiosum

Definition

Molluscum contagiosum is a virus-induced (DNA virus), pearl-like, white to yellowish nodule with a dimple on the top.

Surface Microscopy

There are multiple yellowish-brown keratotic plugs with a whitish halo in the center of the lesion (Fig. 121). The plugs are surrounded by linear and curvilinear vessels, which also slope along the raised edges (red corona). Red dots surrounding the papule are also seen.

Reference

311

Moth-eaten Border

Synonyms

Synonyms for moth-eaten border are Menzies' sign, moth-eaten pigment border, and moth-eaten edge.

Definition

Moth-eaten border is a pigmented lesion with well-defined concave borders, where the pigmentation ends with scalloped ("punched-out") structures (Fig. 122).

Occurrence

Moth-eaten border occurs as flat seborrheic keratoses (mainly on the face), solar lentigo, lentigo maligna, and ephelis (freckle).

References

55; 142; 186; 188; 245; 298

Mountain and Valley Pattern

▶ Fissures and ridges.

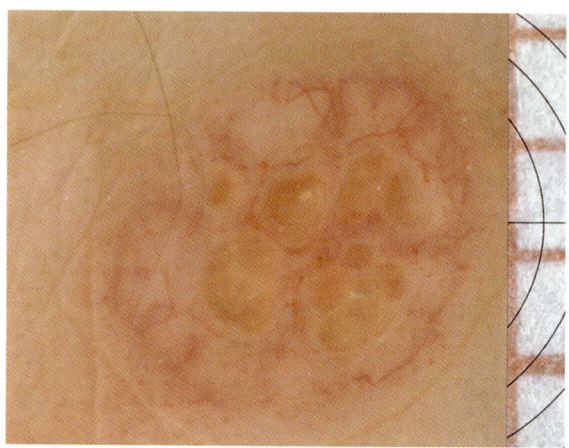

Fig. 121 Molluscum contagiosum shows keratotic plugs surrounded by linear and curvilinear vessels

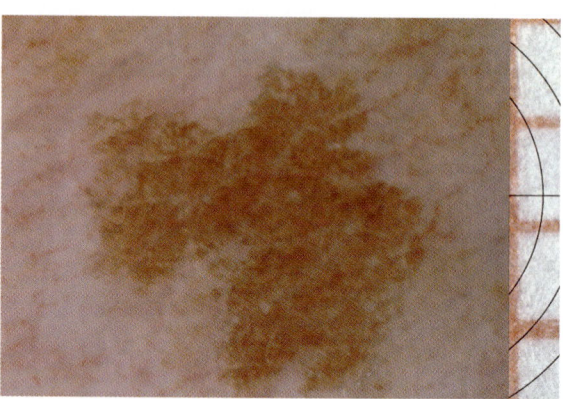

Fig. 122 Ephelis represents a moth-eaten border and a uniform pigmented background (absent brown globules)

Mucosal Melanocytic Macule or Papule

Definition

Mucosal melanocytic macule and papule are benign or malignant melanocytic lesions seen on the lips, glans penis, and female genitalia.

Surface Microscopy

Surface microscopy shows benign lesions are characterized by aggregated light- and dark-brown to slate-gray globules (nests of melanocytes at the dermoepidermal junction), fingerprint patterns, and linear pigmentation interrupted by dots and globules. Tiny punctiform capillaries (normal capillary loops in the center of the dermal papillae) are regularly arranged and usually spread over the entire lesion. Malignant lesions become asymmetric with irregular structures and colors and an abrupt cut-off of the pattern at the periphery. They may show brown-gray to blue-gray pigmentation and slate-gray aggregated granules (melanophages), partly surrounding the vessels, or irregularly distributed globules and dots as well as irregular polymorphous vessels (Figs. 123, 124).

References
62; 298

Mulberry-like Aspect

▶ Target globules.

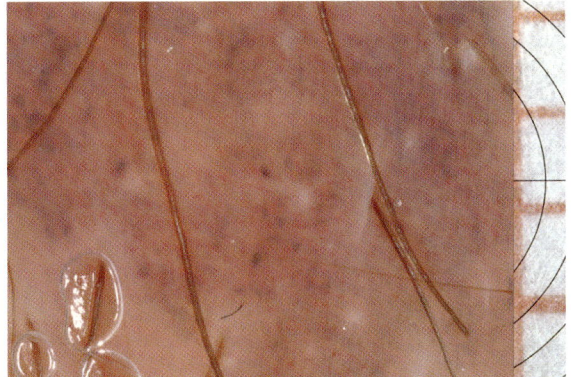

Fig. 123 Compound nevus on the labium pudendi shows multiple slate-gray globules, brown-gray blotches, and regularly arranged red dots (capillaries of the dermal papillae)

Mulberry-like Structure

▶ Target globules.

Multicomponent Pattern

Definition
Multicomponent pattern is a combination of three ore more dermoscopic patterns in the same pigmented lesion (Fig. 125).

Occurrence
Multicomponent pattern occurs as melanocytic nevi (mainly congenital nevi), malignant melanomas (highly suggestive), and recurrent (persistent) nevi.

Reference
82

Multifocal Hyper-/Hypopigmented Pattern

Definition
Multifocal hyper-/hypopigmented pattern is a melanocytic lesion that represents multiple irregularly distributed hyper- and/or hypopigmented zones which suggests dysplastic or malignant changes (Fig. 126). This alteration requires either close follow-up or excision. Other features and criteria for melanocytic alterations may be present.

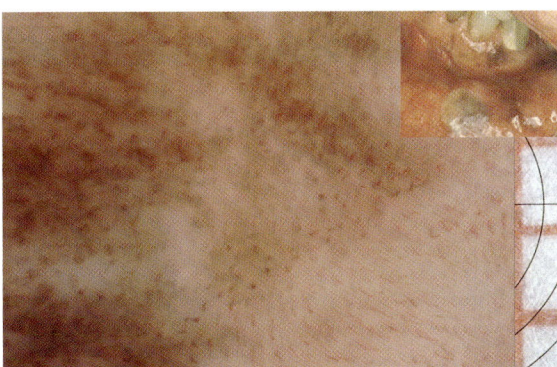

Fig. 124 Mucosal malignant melanoma of the lower lip shows an asymmetric diffuse brown-gray pigmentation, polymorphous capillaries, and a typical gray rim surrounding the dermal papillae

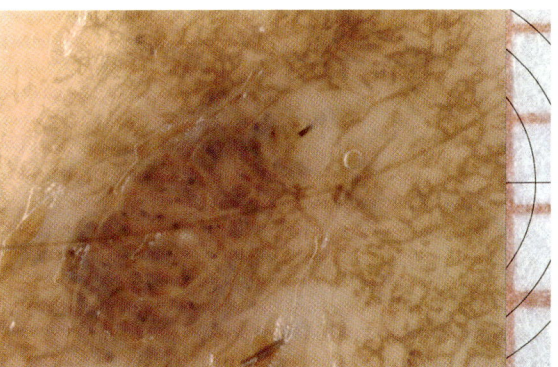

Fig. 125 Congenital nevus shows a multicomponent pattern (reticular, globular, areas of depigmentation and dots)

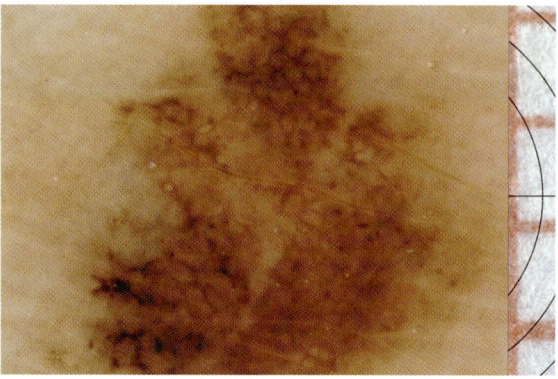

Fig. 126 Compound nevus on the lower leg shows multifocal hyper- and hypopigmented zones

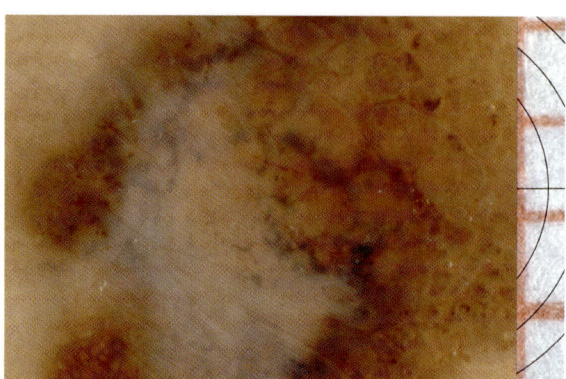

Fig. 127 Compound nevus on the epigastrium shows multiple blue-gray dots (melanin-laden macrophages) within an area of regression

Multiple Blue-gray Dots (Granules)

Synonyms

Synonyms for multiple blue-gray dots are slate-gray granules, blue-gray granules, peppering, and pepper-like area.

Definition

Multiple blue-gray dots melanocytic lesions that represent areas of aggregated and scattered blue-gray to slate-gray granules (melanophages), sometimes in a perivascular arrangement (perivascular melanophages).

Occurrence

Multiple blue-gray dots occur as regressing malignant melanoma (with a specificity of >90% and a sensitivity of >40% for invasive melanoma), lentigo maligna, dysplastic nevus, lichen planus-like keratosis, and regressing benign nevus.

Surface Microscopy

Surface microscopy shows partly aggregated and scattered multiple blue-gray granules ("peppering") commonly seen in association with a hypopigmented scar-like area (regression pattern). Capillaries may be surrounded by aggregates of blue-gray granules (e.g., within a lentigo maligna or an irritated seborrheic keratosis) lacking an association with histological regression (Figs. 127, 128).

Histopathology

Histopathology shows multiple melanin-laden macrophages (melanophages) in the dermis. Associated

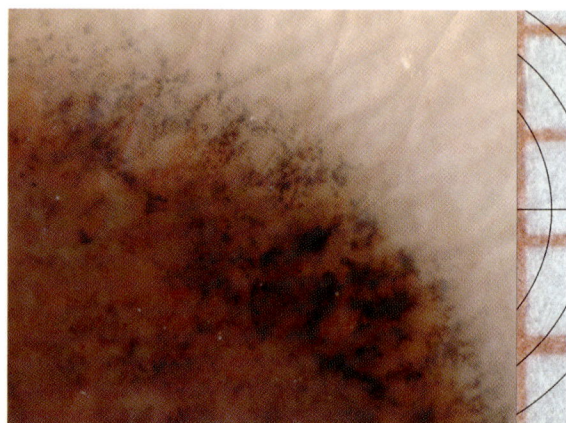

Fig. 128 Unclassified malignant melanoma (Clark level II, Breslow thickness 0.74 mm) in the scapular region. Multiple blue-gray dots in zones of early to intermediate regression are seen as aggregated granules at the border of the lesion

with fibrosis and melanosis in regression are band-like agglomerations of melanophages or tumor cells, teleangiectases, and sparse lymphocytic infiltrates within a thickened papillary dermis.

References

35; 142; 188; 189; 190

Multiple Blue-gray Globules

▶ Globules.

Multiple Blue-gray Ovoid Nests

▶ Gray-black and blue-gray ovoid nests.

Multiple Brown Dots

Definition
These are focal aggregations of dark brown dots (<0.1 mm in diameter) within melanocytic lesions.

Occurrence
Multiple brown dots occur as malignant melanoma (invasive melanomas with a specificity >95% and a sensitivity 30%), rarely seen in benign nevi.

Surface Microscopy
Surface Microscopy shows multiple well-defined aggregations of dark-brown dots (Figs. 129, 130). Scattered or isolated brown dots are a finding of many benign pigmented lesions.

Histopathology
Histopathology shows subcorned or intraepidermal (suprabasal) atypical melanocytes or melanoma cells representing the pagetoid spread of an SSM and occasionally normal melanocytes.

References
184; 189; 190

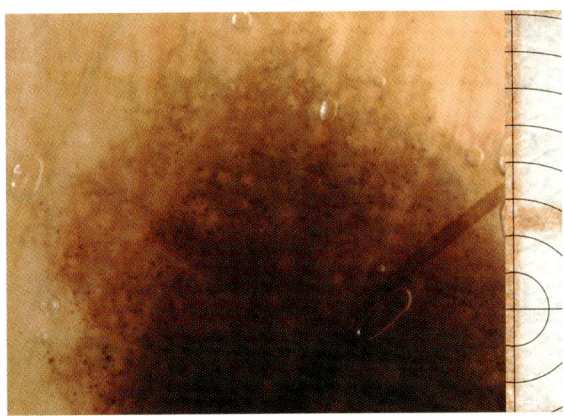

◪ **Fig. 130** Junctional nevus on the trunk shows multiple brown dots spreading throughout the entire lesion

Multiple Brown Globules

▶ Globules.

Multiple Colors

Definition
Melanin agglomerates from the stratum corneum to the mid-dermis and the presence of increased vasculature can lead to multiple colors (Fig. 131). To be a significant predictive feature for melanoma there must be at least five colors from a possible total of six (tan, dark brown, black, gray, red, and blue).

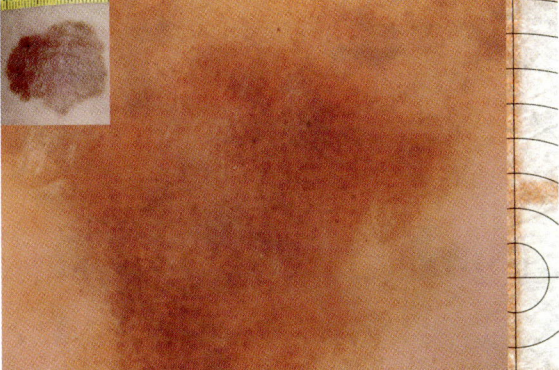

◪ **Fig. 129** Superficial spreading melanoma (Clark level III, Breslow thickness 0.3 mm) on the calf shows multiple focally aggregated brown dots at the periphery of the tumor

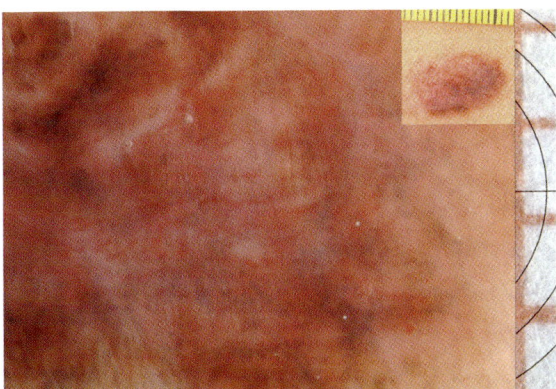

◪ **Fig. 131** This asymmetrically patterned multicolored superficial spreading melanoma has the distinct features of five colors

Occurrence

Multiple colors occur as invasive malignant melanomas (with a specificity of 92% and a sensitivity of 53%).

References

189; 191

Multiple Grayish Patches

▶ Grayish patches.

Nailfold Capillaries, Alterations

Surface Microscopy

The nailfold is the elective site of a capillary disease, characterized by diapedesis bleeding, loss of some capillaries, and capillary sequestration. Histological investigations performed on the living tissue demonstrate how the detached capillaries and the extravasated blood near the epidermis are modified and eliminated at the skin surface (Ehring's rhexis bleeding; Fig. 132). In early stages of scleroderma (systemic sclerosis) the nailfold capillaries embedded into whitish sclerotic tissue are diminished and their diameter is smaller (diameter > 0.03 mm) than normal, except for some intermingled dilated megacapillaries with diameters > 0.05 mm (scleroderma pattern). Occasionally there is some capillary leakage of blood. In dermatomyositis megacapillaries are encountered frequently. Twisted and branching vessels can be observed. Capillary leakages and microhemorrhages within the cuticle occur frequently. In systemic vasculitis and lupus erythema-tosus branching vessels, twisting vessels and microhemorrhages are the most typical findings.

References

48; 89; 90; 91; 161; 176; 194; 196; 244; 247

Nailfold Capillaries, Normal Structure

Definition

Nailfold capillaries of normal structure running parallel to the skin surface nailfold vessels are visible as loops of up to 0.5–2 mm in length.

Surface Microscopy

Juxtaposed to the proximal nail plate, the hairpin-like-shaped capillaries run parallel to the neighboring vessels and the skin surface (Fig. 133). The efferent side of the loop is slightly wider (0.010–0.014 mm) compared with the afferent side (0.008–0.01 mm).

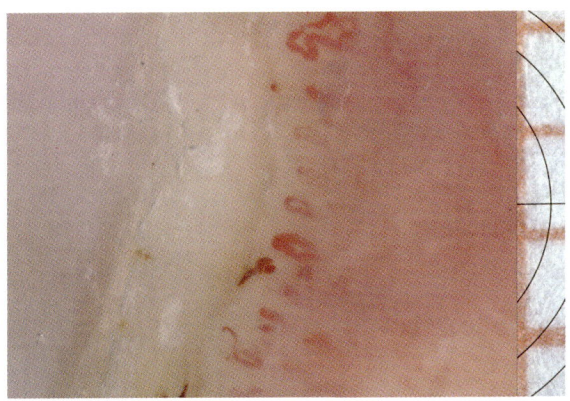

◘ **Fig. 132** Nailfold changes in dermatomyositis shows elongated and ectatic capillary loops, microhemorrhages, and capillary sequestration (Ehring's rhexis bleeding). The dermal plexus is partially visible below the layer of the loops

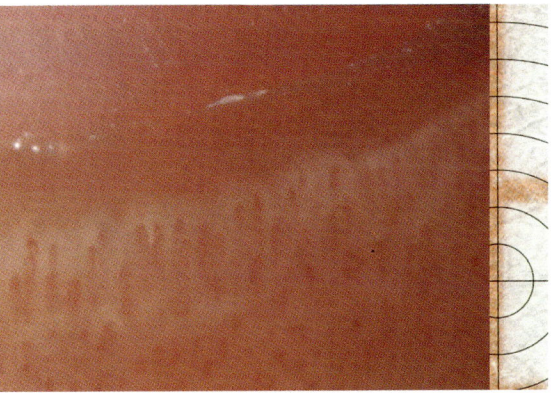

◘ **Fig. 133** Normal nailfold capillaries in a healthy subject (*bars* at intervals of 1 mm)

Reference
161

Negative Network

Synonyms

Synonyms for negative network are inverse network and negative pigment network.

Definition

Melanocytic and non-melanocytic skin lesions with light web- or lace-like network in the background of darker color. This is the mirror image of the "true" pigment network; hence, the term "negative" is applied.

Occurrence

Malignant melanomas (within the group of melanocytic lesions it is a highly specific feature of invasive melanoma, about 95% specificity), dysplastic nevi, Spitz nevi, hemangiomas, hemorrhagic disorders, lymphangiomas, and lymphomas.

Surface Microscopy

A regular or irregular reticular lacy, or mesh-like, light-colored tumor in the background of a darker-colored (pink, red, brown, black) structure (Figs. 134, 135).

Histopathology

Within melanocytic lesions a negative network represents elongated hypomelanotic rete ridges. The dark holes (corresponding to the dermal papillae) are due to pigmented junctional melanocytic nests or other

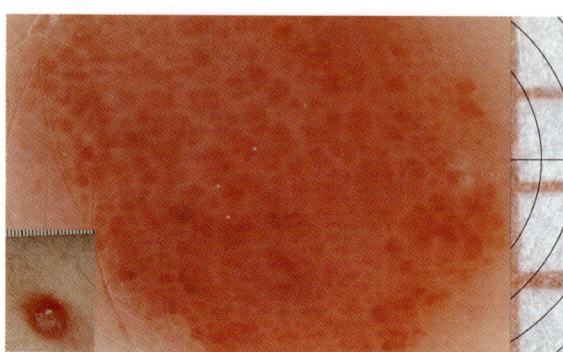

◻ Fig. 135 Unspecified peripheral T-cell lymphoma in the armpit shows a negative network pattern (atypical lymphocytes mixed with erythrocytes within the dermal papillae)

corpuscular elements (e.g., erythrocytes, atypical lymphocytes).

References

12; 47; 188; 190

Neighborhood Sign

Definition

The neighborhood sign is the presence of multiple related neighboring lesions.

Reference

298

Network Holes

Definition

Network holes correspond to the dermal papillae and are relatively hypopigmented, small circular areas that, together with network lines, form a reticular pigment network pattern. In the face the holes correspond to the follicular openings (pseudonetwork).

References

143; 262

Network Irregularity

Synonym

The synonym for network irregularity is prominent and irregular network.

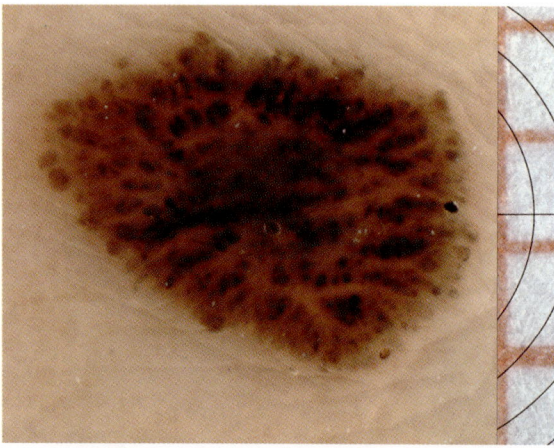

◻ Fig. 134 Spitz nevus on the thorax represents a negative network pattern

Definition

Network irregularity is an architectural disorder of the pigment network in a lesion and represents the overall irregularity of a reticular melanocytic pattern. It may include focal absence or a total loss of the pigment network. A darkly pigmented (prominent) broadened network with irregular-width trabeculae (grids) is usually seen in early melanoma or dysplastic nevi, and in addition there is often an abrupt network edge. Uniform pseudobroadened networks created by dilated follicular openings are often seen within benign nevi, freckles, lentigenes, and actinic keratoses on the face.

References

143; 188; 305

Network Lines

Definition

Network lines correspond to the rete ridges and are short linear brown streaks that, together with network holes, form the reticular pigment network of the skin. In the face and some other regions the network lines may correspond to interfollicular regions (pseudonetwork).

Reference

143

Network Patches, Dark

Definition

Dark network patches are melanocytic lesions with relatively darker network lines compared with the average network line darkness within the lesion. There are subtle histological differences in overall melanin content of the epidermis.

Reference

143

Network Patches, Light

Definition

Light network patches are melanocytic lesions with regions of relatively hypopigmented network lines compared with the average network coloration. This phenomenon is due to subtle histological differences in overall melanin content of the epidermis.

Reference

143

Nevus Cell

Synonyms

Synonyms for nevus cell are nevocyte and nevomelanocyte.

Definition

Nevus cells are closely related to melanocytes, which also originate from the neural crest, and they may or may not synthesize and contain melanin pigment. They are usually small, round, or oval cells with variable-size nuclei and pale cytoplasm, usually without dendrites. The nucleus is larger than that of normal melanocytes. In contrast to the melanocytes, they are not diffusely distributed in the basal layer of the epidermis but form localized nests (strand or in single file) at the dermoepidermal junction or in the dermis.

Nevus Spilus

Synonyms

Synonyms for nevus spilus are congenital speckled lentiginous nevus, congenital zosteriform speckled lentiginous nevus, and segmental lentiginosis.

Definition

Nevus spilus comprise a combination of the café-au-lait spot and the nevus cell nevus with sharply demarcated, light-brown background pigmentation in which numerous darker brownish freckle-like macules are

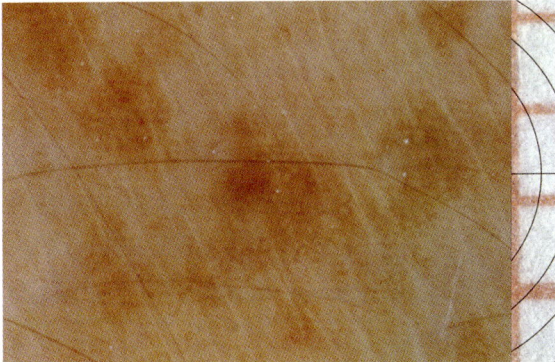

◘ **Fig. 136** Nevus spilus consists of multiple light-brown network patches

scattered. In segmental lentiginosis there are often associated neurological abnormalities.

Histopathology

The light-brown zone consists of increased basal layer pigment with elongation of rete ridges (Fig. 136). The darker areas are melanocytic nevi of the junctional or compound type.

References

118; 148; 220; 289; 298

Nodular Malignant Melanoma

Definition

Nodular malignant melanoma is a malignant melanocytic lesion that has primarily a vertical growth phase and lacks of significant intraepidermal tumor growth beyond the margins of the invasive dermal component.

Surface Microscopy

Typically there are mainly features associated with thick melanoma: blue-white veil; atypical vascular patterns (irregularly distributed dotted vessels, linear–irregular and polymorphous vessels); asymmetric pigmentation pattern; regression patterns; and milky-red globules or areas with irregular extensions. Ulcerations with bleeding are common.

Histopathology

Numerous atypical melanocytes singly and in nests are seen at the dermoepidermal junction as well as throughout the epidermis (Fig. 137). Confluent nests

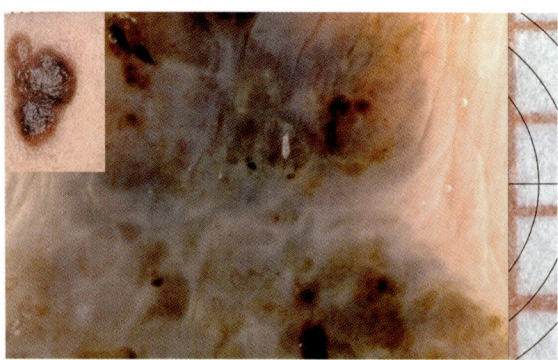

☐ **Fig. 137** Nodular melanoma (Clark level IV, Breslow thickness 1.85 mm) on the upper arm shows a blue-white veil, multiple colors, irregularly distributed black dots, irregular vessels, and an oval blood lake

and sheets of melanocytes without maturation invade the dermis. The dermal component shows extensive pleiomorphism with numerous abnormal mitosis figures. There is a minimal intraepidermal involvement at the periphery of the tumor.

References

7; 16; 188; 191; 298

Non-specific Pattern

Definition

A "non-specific" pattern refers to a combination of findings which do not have specific diagnostic implications. The term should be used if a pigmented lesion does not exhibit one of the following patterns: reticular pattern; globular pattern; cobblestone pattern; homogeneous pattern; starburst pattern; parallel pattern (palms and soles); and multicomponent pattern.

Reference

82

Normal Skin Surface

The normal, finely furrowed skin surface of the trunk and the largest portions of the extremities consist of raised, cushion-like fields which are rhombic, trapezoid, or triangular in shape (measuring up to 0.8 mm in length). The highest points within these fields show delicate punctiform or thread-like vessels which represent capillary loops that go out from the superficial dermal plexus to supply singly the dermal papillae (Fig. 132). Transepidermal water loss causes distortion of the skin topography to form parallel striae, associated with a loss of turgor of the normally plump, cushioned surface. The palms and soles have a particular architecture which consists of parallel ridges and furrows. The ridges, i.e., papillary ridges, correspond to the crista superficialis and the sulcus correspond to the sulcus superficialis. Openings of the eccrine pores (eccrine ducts) are seen as whitish dots regularly arranged in the center of the papillary ridges with a space of 0.4–0.5 mm. The diameter of the non-pigmented dot (acrosyringeum), including a whitish halo, is 0.08 mm. Diameters of the ostia vary between 0.02 and 0.09 mm.

References

124; 256; 262

O

Old-age Spot

► Solar lentigo.

Orthokeratosis

Orthokeratosis is formation of an anuclear scaly layer of the epidermis caused by normal keratinization with complete catabolism of the nuclei.

Ovoid Blood Lakes

Synonym
Synonyms are microscopic ovoid blood lakes and blood lakes.

Definition
Ovoid blood lakes are microscopic blood lakes that represent microhemorrhages next to aneurysmatic vessels.

Occurrence
Ovoid blood lakes occur as malignant melanocytic and malignant epithelial tumors.

References
261; 262

Ovoid Nests

► Gray-black and blue-gray ovoid nests.

Pagetoid Malignant Melanoma

▶ Superficial spreading melanoma.

Palms and Soles

▶ Dermatoglyphics.
▶ Normal skin.
▶ Parallel furrow pattern.

Papillary Layer

▶ Stratum papillare.

Papillomatous
or Dome-shaped Melanocytic Nevus

Synonym
The synonym is Unna's nevus.

Definition
These lesions are mostly exophytic and soft melanocytic lesions usually with a lobulated border and numerous convex structures.

Surface Microscopy
The central area has a large cobblestone-like papillomatous portion with asymmetrical variations in distribution of slate-gray to dark brown pigment (Fig. 138). If a vascular pattern is present, it is characterized by comma-shaped, arciform, and linear vessels. There may also be a junctional or compound component with a pigment network or branched streaks.

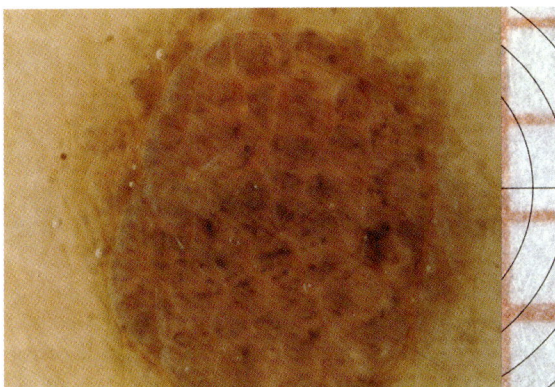

■ **Fig. 138** Papillomatous melanocytic nevus demonstrates a cobblestone-like pattern and a lobulated periphery with convex border

Histopathology
They are characterized by being more exophytic than endophytic in most instances, mostly intradermal, and associated with a pattern of nests, cords, and strands of melanocytes and neurocytes within the exophytic papillary dermis.

Reference
5

Parakeratosis

Incomplete or qualitatively abnormal keratinization with retention of nuclei in the keratinocytes of the stratum corneum of the epidermis. It is commonly observed in many scaling dermatoses such as psoriasis and subacute or chronic dermatitis. The stratum granulosum is largely absent or diminished in psoriasis. Using surface microscopy, parakeratosis without an associated hypergranulosis may cause more transparency of the epidermis.

Parallel Furrow Pattern

Definition

Parallel furrow pattern consists of pigmented skin of the palms and soles with light-brown to black lines (striped streaks) corresponding to pigmentation within the parallel furrows of the surface skin markings (sulcus superficialis), and running parallel to the papillary ridges (Fig. 139).

Occurrence

The presence of a parallel pattern with accentuation of pigmentation along the sulcus is usually associated with benign volar and plantar nevi.

Surface Microscopy

Melanocytes in benign lesions tend to concentrate about the crista limitans, which lies beneath the sulcus superficialis. One may see a single line of pigmentation within each furrow (type 1A), a single dotted line (type 1B), a line of pigmentation on each side of the sulcus (type 1C: double-line variant), or a dotted line on each side of the furrow (type 1D: double dotted-line variant). On top of the papillary tips the eccrine sweat gland ostia are lined up parallel to the linear pigmentation.

Histopathology

Individual melanocytes or nests of nevus cells are mostly found in crista profunda limitans (epidermal rete ridges underlying the surface sulci).

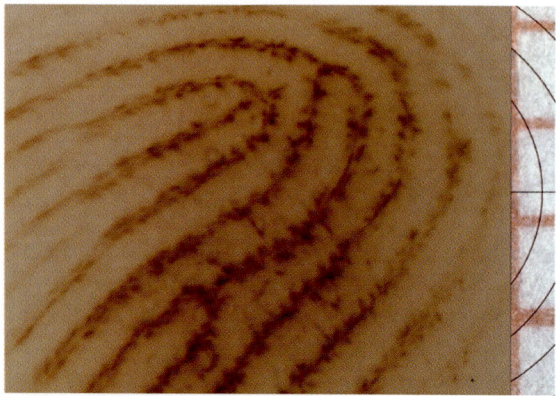

◘ **Fig. 139** Melanocytic nevus on the plantar side of the first toe shows a parallel furrow pattern, double-lined variant

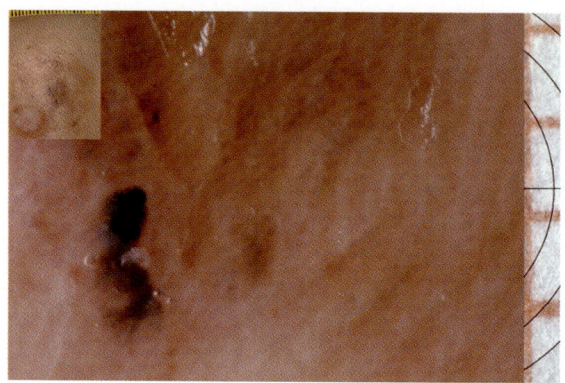

◘ **Fig. 140** Mainly hypomelanotic acrolentiginous plantar-warts-like melanoma on the sole (Clark level IV, Breslow thickness 4.9 mm) demonstrates an indistinct parallel ridge pattern (in the right and upper part of the lesion) and gray-brown to gray-black irregular globules up to 0.8 mm in diameter (in the *left* part)

References

110; 240

Parallel Ridge Pattern

Definition

Parallel ridge pattern (PRP) comprises melanocytic lesions of the palms and soles with band-like pigmentation along the ridges. The surface sulci are often spared from pigmentation (Fig. 140).

Occurrence

The presence of pigmentation along the ridges and/or the presence of irregular diffuse pigmentation are highly suggestive of malignant melanoma. It is rarely seen in benign nevi. The PRP is an important feature in detecting acrolentiginous melanoma, with a sensitivity of 86% and a specificity of 99%.

Histopathology

On histopathology PRP shows melanocytes which proliferate mainly within the crista profunda intermedia.

References

110; 239; 240

Parallel Striae

► Corticosteroid side effects.

Patchy Network Pattern

Definition
Patchy network pattern is a melanocytic nevus with islands of relatively uniform network that are separated by areas of structureless background (indicative of a benign nature of the lesion; Fig. 141).

Reference
304

Peppering

▶ Multiple blue-gray dots.

Perifollicular Circular Gray-blue/Gray-black Pigmentation

▶ Perifollicular pigment changes.

Perifollicular Pigment Changes

Synonyms
Synonyms for perifollicular pigment changes are gray-black perifollicular pigmentation, perifollicular gray-blue circular pigmentation, perifollicular rim of hyperpigmentation, and asymmetric pigmented follicular openings.

Definition
Perifollicular pigment changes are hypopigmentation or hyperpigmentation that occurs around the hair follicles.

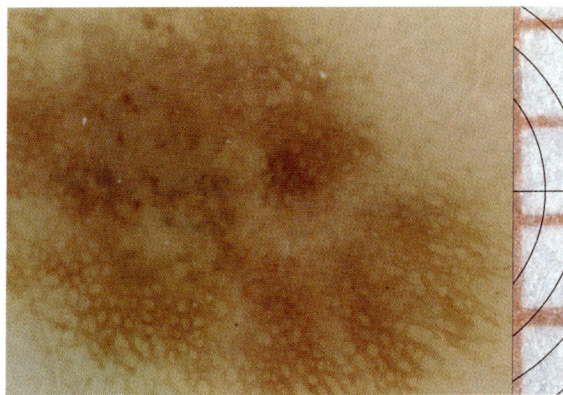

Fig. 141 Compound nevus with a patchy network pattern

Occurrence
Gray-black or gray-blue perifollicular pigmentation is suggestive of melanoma, particularly lentigo maligna or lentigo maligna melanoma, and in some cases congenital nevi.

Surface Microscopy
There is an alteration of the perifollicular pigment pattern manifested as dark-brown to black asymmetrically distributed in a lacy to rhomboid pattern.

Histopathology
The pigmentary changes correspond to the perifollicular extension of atypical melanocytes, both interfollicularly and in the deeper aspects of the hair follicles.

References
174; 188

Perifollicular Rim of Hyperpigmentation

▶ Perifollicular pigment changes.

Peripheral Black Dots

Synonym
The synonym is peripheral brown/black dots.

Definition
Peripheral black dots are melanocytic lesions with distinctly black or dark brown dots (<0.1 mm in diameter) near the border of the lesion.

Occurrence
Peripheral black dots occur as malignant melanoma (specificity >90%, sensitivity >40%) and dysplastic nevi (usually central black dots).

Surface Microscopy
Black dots, localized at or near the edge of the lesion, usually represent malignant melanocytes found at or near the stratum corneum (Fig. 142).

Histopathology
Histopathology shows focal collections of melanin within the superficial layer of the stratum corneum or stratum granulosum, mainly arising from pagetoid spread of heavily pigmented atypical melanocytes.

References

189; 190; 298; 323

Peripheral Brown Dots

▶ Peripheral black dots.

Peripheral Erythema

▶ Red corona.

Peripheral Hypopigmented Pattern

Definition

Peripheral hypopigmented pattern is a melanocytic lesion representing peripheral hypopigmented, partly structureless areas that suggest dysplastic or malignant changes (Fig. 143). That alteration requires either close follow-up or excision. Other typical features and criteria for melanocytic lesions may be present.

Peripheral Network with Central Hyperpigmentation

Definition

This is a melanocytic nevus characterized by a peripheral network associated with a blotchy area of central hyperpigmentation (usually indicative of a benign nature of the lesion; Fig. 144).

Reference

304

Peripheral Network with Central Hypopigmentation

Definition

This is a melanocytic nevus characterized by a peripheral network associated with a central area that is relatively structureless and less pigmented than the periphery (indicative of a benign nature of the lesion; Fig. 145).

Reference

304

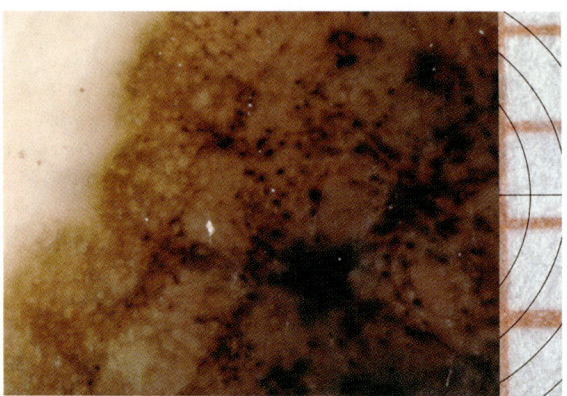

Fig. 142 Superficial spreading melanoma (Clark level IV, Breslow thickness 4.4 mm) shows multiple black dots near the edge of the lesion

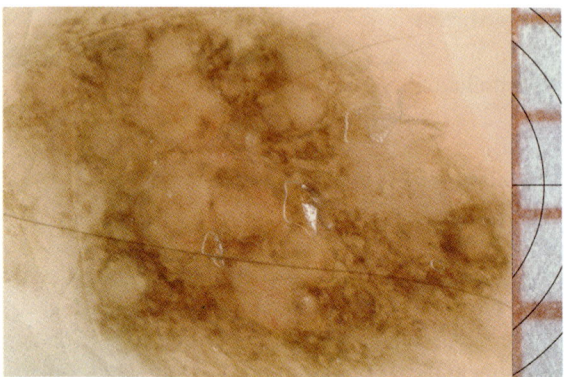

Fig. 143 Compound nevus on the scapular region shows multiple irregularly distributed round to polygonal hypopigmented areas at the periphery of the lesion and in the center

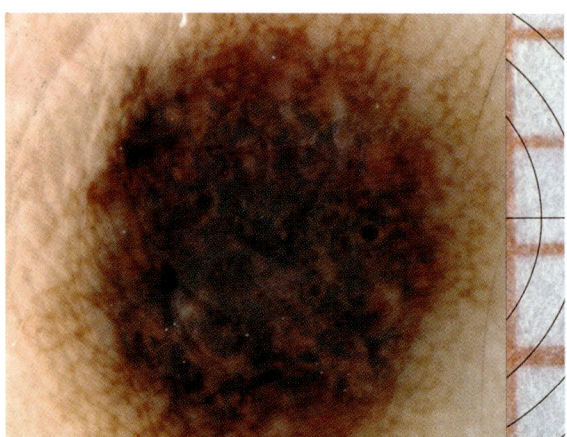

Fig. 144 Atypical mole with a peripheral network pattern and central hyperpigmemtation (central regression zone)

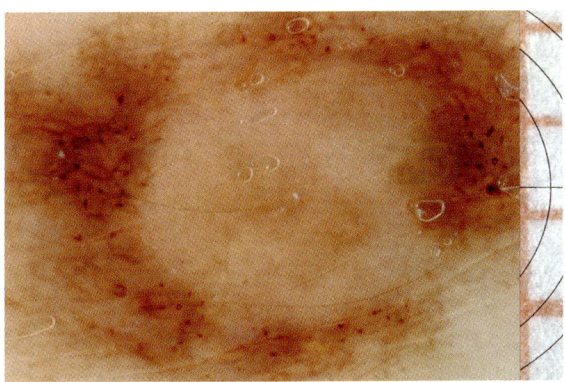

Fig. 145 Compound nevus with a peripheral network pattern and central hypopigmentation

Perivascular Melanophages

▶ Multiple blue-gray dots.

Persistent Nevi

▶ Recurrent (persistent) nevi.

Pigment Globules

▶ Globules.

Pigment Network

Definition

Pigment network is a honeycomb (grid-like) network of the skin surface that consists of pigmented "lines" (corresponding with the rete ridges) and hypopigmented "holes" (corresponding with the tips of the dermal papillae). It is formed by melanocytes and pigmented keratinocytes at the basal layer.

Occurrence

Pigment network occurs as ephelis, solar lentigo, junctional and compound nevi (gradually ending network edge), dysplastic nevi (irregular-width grids and abrupt network edge), or malignant melanomas.

Surface Microscopy

The epidermal projections of the pigmented reticulation, due to melanocytes and melanin in the keratino-cytes, represent the rete ridges constituting the grids of the network. The relatively hypomelanotic holes in the network correspond to tips of the dermal papillae and the overlying suprapapillary plates of the epidermis. A typical network is relatively uniform, regularly meshed, homogeneous in color, and usually thins out at the periphery (gradually ending network edge; Fig. 146). If the rete ridges are short or less pigmented, the pigment network may not be visible. The pigment network on the palms and soles can be divided into the parallel furrow pattern, the lattice-like pattern, and the fibrillar/filamentous pattern.

Histopathology

Melanin pigment is localized either in basal keratinocytes, or in melanocytes along the dermoepidermal junction.

References

12; 21; 142; 143; 180; 186; 211; 279; 298; 323

Pigmentation

▶ Color changes.
▶ Melanin pigmentation.

Pigmented Hairy Epidermal Nevus

▶ Melanosis neviformis.

Pigmented Skin Lesions on Palms and Soles

▶ Parallel furrow pattern.

Fig. 146 A typical network of the well-pigmented areola of a mammary gland in a 38-year-old woman

Pilosebaceous Unit

▶ Follicular plug and opening.

Pinpoint Vessels

▶ Dotted vessels.

Pityriasis Lichenoides

▶ Purpuric lesions.

Plaster-of-Paris-like Lacunae

Synonym

The synonym for plaster-of-paris-like lacunae is Alabaster gypseous lacunae.

Definition

Alabaster-colored gypseous lacunae are abnormal small grayish or whitish-opaque spaces (cavities) between the dermal layers or between cellular elements of the dermis of melanocytic lesions.

Occurrence

They occur as malignant melanomas (a specificity of 95% and a sensitivity of 30% for advanced invasive melanoma) and recurrent nevi.

Surface Microscopy

Surface microscopy shows round to elongated or polygonal spaces resembling punched-out cavities filled with grayish or whitish-opaque gypsum-like material (replacement fibrosis; Fig. 147). Remnants of pigmented rete ridges may overlay the fibrous structures of the replacement fibrosis.

Histopathology

Histopathology shows circumscribed formations of fibrous tissue replacing tumor cells within the lower stratum papillare near the border of the stratum reticulare.

References

231; 257

PN

▶ Pigment network.

Polymorphic Angiectatic Base Pattern

Definition

This is a vascular pattern of melanocytic lesions that corresponds to a base pattern of polymorphic ectatic blood vessels and/or sacciform dilated capillaries (aneurysms; Fig. 148).

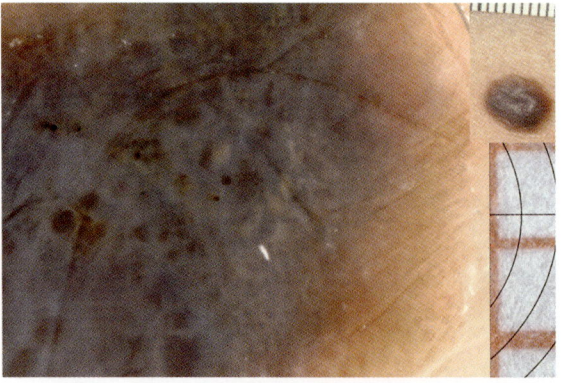

Fig. 147 Superficial spreading melanoma on the lower leg (Clark level IV, Breslow thickness 2.22 mm) presents grayish opaque lacunae in the center of the lesion

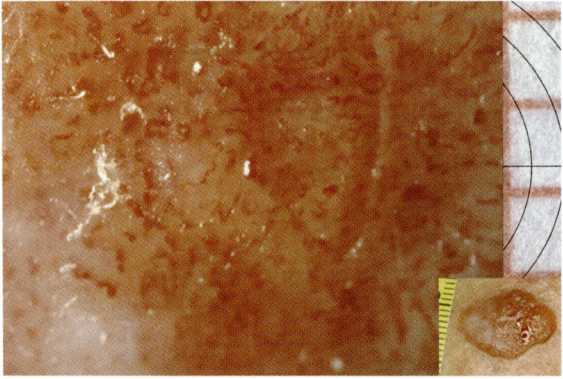

Fig. 148 Nodular melanoma on the scapular region (Clark level IV, Breslow thickness 3.01 mm) shows polymorphic and aneurysmatic blood vessels not identifiably associated with the normal dermal papillary vascular pattern

Occurrence

Polymorphic angiectatic base pattern occurs as malignant melanomas, cutaneous melanoma metastases (with a specificity of 98% and a sensitivity of 43.3%), and occasionally benign nevi (without significant variations in the caliber and shape of the blood vessels).

Surface Microscopy

Malignant neocapillaries spreading throughout the entire lesion are partially saccular dilated (aneurysms) and do not correspond to the normal dermal vascularization. Numerous newly formed convolutions of dilated capillaries can be seen. Some polymorphic capillaries mimic Greek minuscules.

References

251; 252; 261; 262; 263

Polymorphous Vessels

▶ Irregular vessels.

Polypoid Malignant Melanoma

Definition

Polypoid malignant melanoma is a peduncular variant of the nodular malignant melanoma.

Surface Microscopy

The main pattern consists of milky-red or blue-red areas (vascularized amelanotic or hypomelanotic tumor cell complexes), polymorphous vessels, and/or surface vessels resembling irregular hairpin-like-shaped capillaries. Often there are remnants of the network at the edge of the lesion.

Histopathology

Histopathology shows a polypoid configuration and growth pattern of atypical spindle-shaped and epithelioid melanocytes in sheets and nests extending deep into the dermis (Fig. 149).

References

193; 298

Polythelia

▶ Supernumerary nipple.

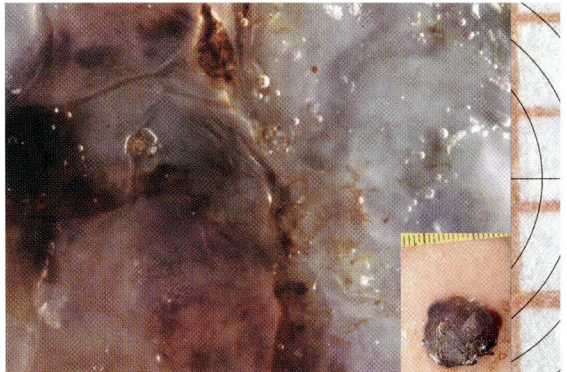

◻ **Fig. 149** Polypoid malignant melanoma on the upper arm (Clark level III, Breslow thickness 5.23 mm) represents vascularized blue-red areas

Porokeratosis

Definition

Porokeratosis consists of solitary or multiple lesions which begin as a small papule with a central horny peg which eventually develop into a macule or flat-topped papule with a distinct peripheral scaly rim. The histological investigation reveals a multifocal circumscribed impairment of epidermal differentiation resulting in an inwardly oriented parakeratotic rim (coronoid lamella) at the periphery of the lesion.

Surface Microscopy

A characteristic raised, hyperkeratotic border is surrounded by ectatic and dotted vessels (Fig. 150).

References

81; 311

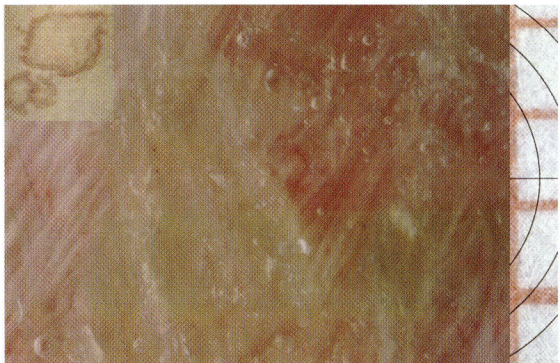

◻ **Fig. 150** Porokeratosis of Mibelli shows a hyperkeratotic border surrounded by ectatic vessels

Prickle Cell Layer

▶ Stratum spinosum.

Proliferation Hyperkeratosis

▶ Hyperkeratosis.

Prominent and Irregular Network

▶ Network irregularity.

PRP

▶ Parallel ridge pattern.

Pseudobroadened Network

▶ Broadened network.
▶ Network irregularity.

Pseudofollicular Openings

▶ Comedo-like openings.

Pseudohorncysts

Synonyms
Synonyms for pseudohorncysts are milia-like cysts and pseudohorn-like cysts.

Definition
Pseudohorncysts are circular white-yellow, opalescent round areas within the body of a lesion. The size varies from 0.1 to 1 mm in diameter.

Occurrence
Pseudohorncysts occur as lentigo senilis, seborrheic keratosis (multiple), compound or dermal nevus, papillomatous melanocytic nevus, congenital nevus, basal cell carcinoma (individual), fibroepithelioma (Pinkus tumor), and malignant melanoma (individual).

Histopathology
Histopathology shows intraepidermal keratin cysts (Fig. 151).

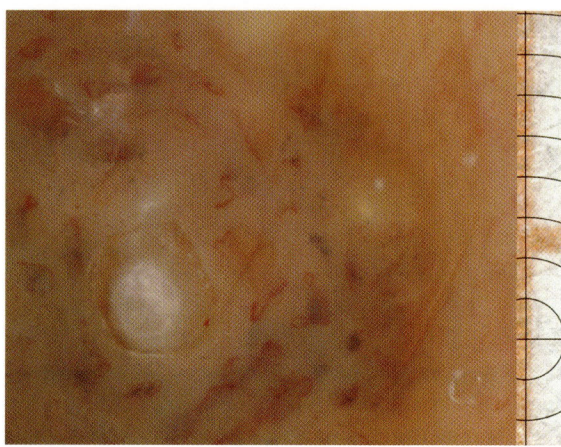

◘ Fig. 151 A pseudohorn cyst in an acanthotic seborrheic keratosis

References
31; 142; 184; 186; 188; 271; 298

Pseudohorn-like Cysts

▶ Pseudohorncysts.

Pseudomelanoma

▶ Recurrent (persistent) nevi.

Pseudonetwork

Definition
A pseudonetwork is formed by the close association of follicular openings in the background of hyperpigmentation, mainly manifested on the head and neck area of adult skin. It is characterized by a broad mesh and holes created by numerous pigment-free terminal and vellus hair follicular orifices as well as the openings of sweat glands (Figs. 152, 153).

Surface Microscopy
A characteristic pigmentation is often not present on the facial skin of adults. Since the rete ridges are flat to absent, there is no histological constituent to form a primary pigment network. Instead, the network-like structures are produced by the close association of the openings of skin appendages superimposed on pigmented areas.

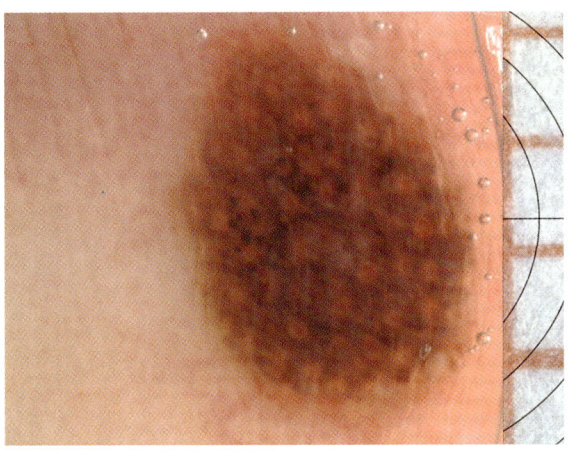

🔲 **Fig. 152** Compound nevus on the earlobe shows a typical pseudonetwork

Occurrence

Pseudopods are almost never found in benign lesions, except in Spitz nevi (with a uniform circumferential position of the pseudopods). They represent the characteristically radial growth phase of superficial spreading melanoma (with a specificity of 97% and a sensitivity of 23% for invasive melanomas).

Surface Microscopy

Tan-to-black pigmented asymmetric and irregular branched streaks extend into the adjacent skin. The kinked finger-like peripheral extensions may have small knobs at their tips, and are either connected to the pigment network or directly connected to the main tumor body. In contrast to radial streaming, they are not linear but irregularly curved or bended.

🔲 **Fig. 153** Compound nevus on the forehead of a young man shows a primary pigment network (in the *left* and *lower* portion of the lesion) in combination with a pseudonetwork (in the *upper* and *right* portion)

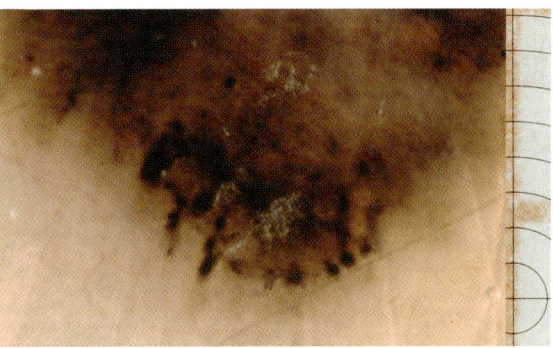

🔲 **Fig. 154** Superficial spreading melanoma on the thigh (Clark level II, Breslow thickness 0.54 mm). It represents pseudopods at the lesion's margin

References

12; 271

Pseudopods

Synonyms

Synonyms for pseudopods are irregular pigmentary extensions and slate-gray pseudopods.

Definition

Pseudopods are melanocytic lesions with morphologically highly variable kinked or bulbous finger-like extensions of brown, black, or slate-gray pigment at the periphery (Figs. 154, 155).

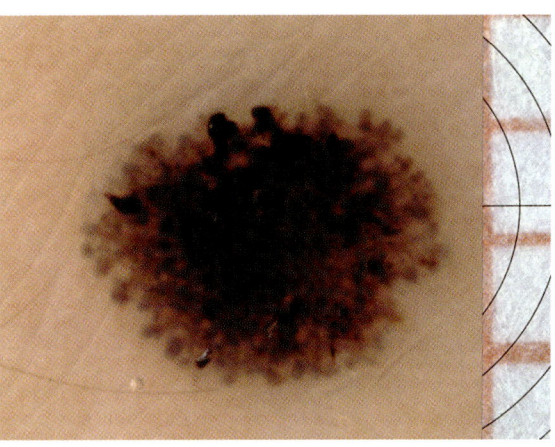

🔲 **Fig. 155** Spitz nevus on the lower leg shows uniform circumferential pseudopods at the margin

Histopathology

Pseudopods correspond to intraepidermal or junctional confluent radial nests of melanocytes.

References

82; 142; 183; 184; 186; 188; 189; 213

Pseudostreaks

Definition

Pseudostreaks are an aggregation of pigment within the sulci of folded surfaces in papillomatous skin lesions (e.g., papillomatous nevi, seborrheic keratoses; Fig. 156). They are usually thicker than ordinary, true branched streaks with or without additional short branches.

Reference

298

Pseudotrabeculae of Blue-gray Granules

▶ Pseudotrabeculae of melanophages.

Pseudotrabeculae of Melanophages

▶ Annular–granular pattern.

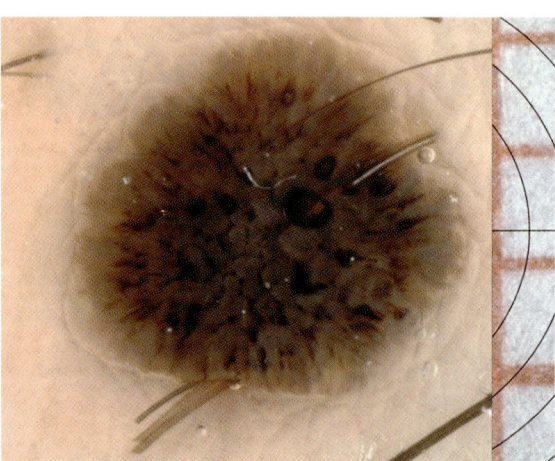

◘ Fig. 156 Pigmented seborrheic keratosis shows radially arranged pseudostreaks at the periphery and reticular pseudostreaks in the center of the lesion. Note the multiple comedo-like openings with black rims

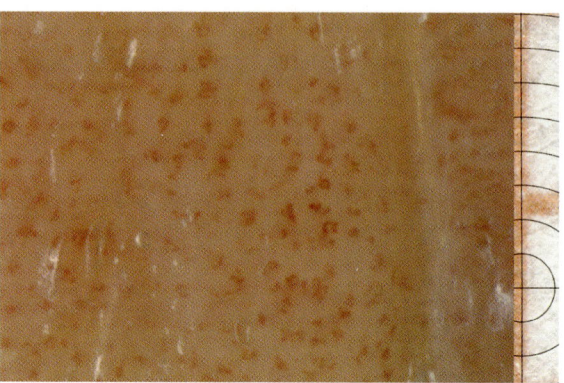

◘ Fig. 157 Erythematous plaque–psoriasis shows regularly distributed convoluted papillary angiectasias. The subpapillary plexus is not visible (due to psoriasiform hyperplasia)

Psoriasis and Spongiotic Dermatitis

Surface Microscopy

The plaque–psoriasis erythematosus, spongiotic psoriasiform dermatitis, and seborrheic dermatitis reveal regularly distributed interfollicular red globules, i.e., papillary angiectasias which consists of convoluted dilated capillary loops, the so-called cotton-ball phenomenon (Fig. 157). Perivascular areas generally show pink- to red-colored patches. Superficial microhemorrhages are often associated with more exudative forms.

References

104; 237; 308; 311

Psoriatic Oil Spot

▶ Brown background, nail unit.

Purpuric Lesions

Surface Microscopy

Senile purpura show large, irregularly shaped homogeneous purpuric patches devoid of definite rounded structures. Vasculitis, pigmented purpuric dermatoses. or acute pityriasis lichenoides reveal purpuric dots/globules within orange-brown patches and surrounding these structures (Fig. 158).

Reference

311

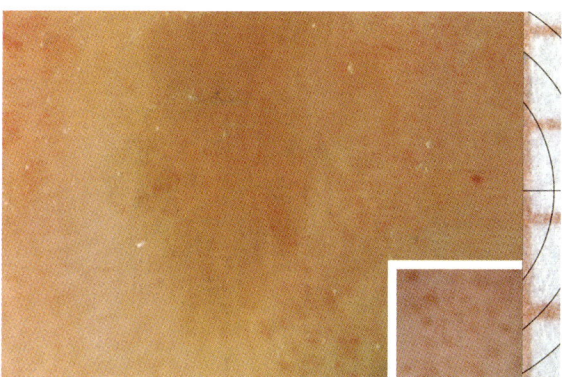

◘ **Fig. 158** Acute pityriasis lichenoides on the thoracic region represents purpuric dots and globules within orange-brown patches and surrounding them

Rabinovitz Sign

► Spoke-wheel-like structures.

Radial Streaming

Synonyms

Synonyms for radial streaming are streaks, irregular or regular streaks, and digitiform extrusions.

Definition

Radial streaming consists of a melanocytic lesion with radially and asymmetrically or symmetrically arranged parallel linear extensions of the pigment network at the edges.

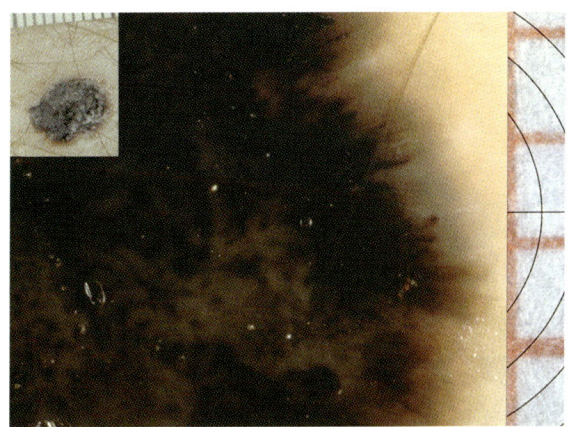

Fig. 159 Superficial spreading melanoma on the lower leg (Clark level III, Breslow thickness 0.73 mm). The *inset* shows a typical radial streaming at the margin

Occurrence

Radial streaming occurs as radial growth phase of malignant melanoma (irregular streaks with a specificity of 96% and a sensitivity of 18%), and Spitz nevus (regular streaks with a symmetrical arrangement).

Surface Microscopy

Surface microscopy shows dark-brown to black radially and symmetrically or asymmetrically arranged parallel linear and tapered pigmentary extensions occurring at the edges of, or occasionally within, the lesion (Figs. 159, 160). It may be a very subtle feature in some melanomas, often in association with a diffuse pigmented gray-blue background.

Histopathology

There are confluent radially orientated nests of pigmented melanocytes within the epidermis and the dermoepidermal junction, with a prominent transepidermal melanin extension.

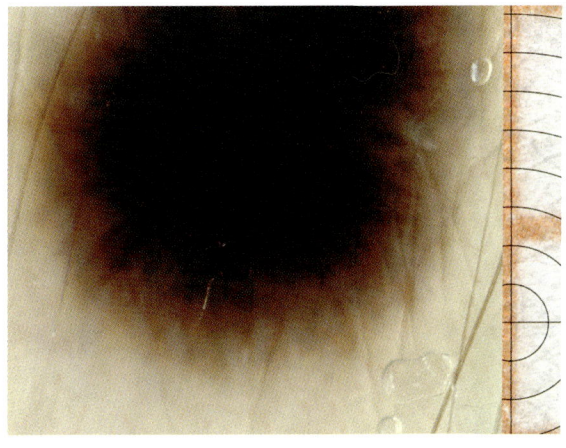

Fig. 160 Spitz Nevus with a radial streaming at the margin

References

21; 82; 142; 184; 186; 189

Radial Symmetrical Streaks

▶ Starburst pattern.

Recurrent (Persistent) Nevus

Synonyms

Synonyms for recurrent nevus are pseudomelanoma and recurrent melanocytic nevus.

Definition

Recurrent nevus is recurrence of pigmentation that appears after an incomplete excision of a benign melanocytic nevus, usually within 6 months. The persistent nevi may resemble flat melanomas.

Surface Microscopy

The features include bizarre pigmentations, atypical pigment networks, asymmetric homogeneous or multi-component patterns, regression structures, and blue-gray or red colors. There may be irregular streaks, black dots, or globules (Figs. 161, 162). The pigment is usually confined to the center of the white scar. The entire scar may be surrounded by a light-brown halo.

Histopathology

There are minimally atypical melanocytes in singles or nests along the dermoepidermal junction. Melanocytes may be present in the epidermis, epithelial structures of adnexa, and, occasionally, in the uppermost part of the dermis. Fibrosis with increased vascularity can be seen beneath the basal layer. There may be residual dermal nevus cells deeper in the dermis.

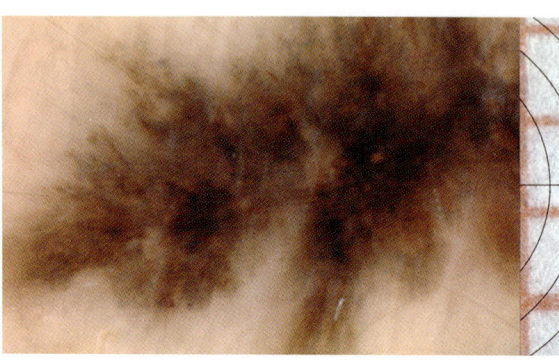

◘ **Fig. 162** Recurrent compound nevus on the scapular region which reveals many features including irregular streaks, slate-gray dots (melanophages), globules, and regression structures (peppering)

References

5; 75; 116; 117; 118; 150; 169; 171; 175; 272

Red Corona

Synonyms

Synonyms for red corona are peripheral erythema and hairpin-like-shaped corona.

Definition

Red corona consists of dotted, hairpin-like-shaped, or polymorphous vessels that surround the lesion (Fig. 163).

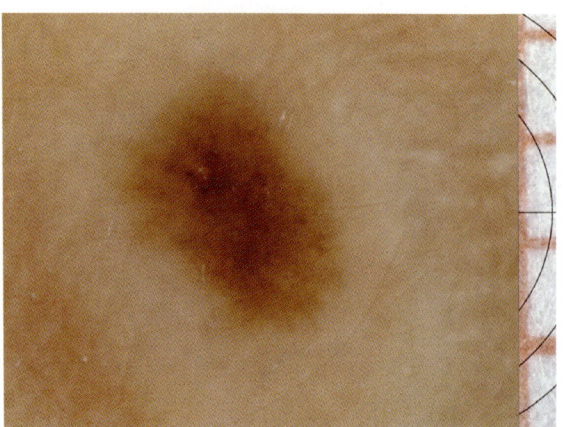

◘ **Fig. 161** Recurrent compound nevus within the white scar on the back. The scar is surrounded by a light-brown halo

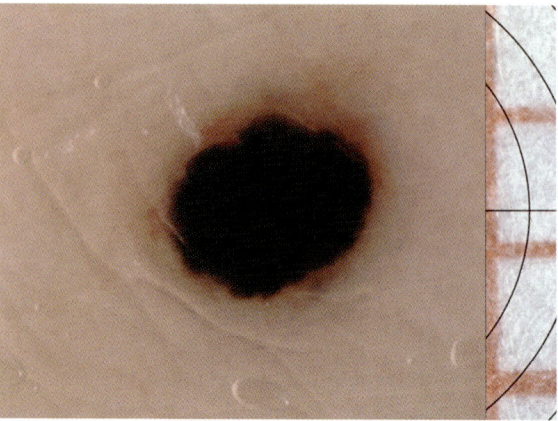

◘ **Fig. 163** Cutaneous malignant melanoma metastasis on the thigh shows a red corona surrounding the border

Occurrence

Red corona occur as malignant melanomas, malignant melanoma metastases, and molluscum contagiosum (linear vessels sloping along the raised edge).

Histopathology

Histopathology shows dilated blood vessels in the papillary dermis at the periphery of the lesion.

References

160; 261

Red Lagoons

▶ Lacunae.

Red Parallel Ridge Pattern

▶ Black heel.

Red-blue Areas

▶ Lacunae.

Reed Nevus

▶ Spitz nevus.

Regressing Malignant Melanoma

▶ Melanoma with marked regression.

Regression Pattern

Synonyms

Synonyms for regression pattern are regression structures, white and blue areas, regressive areas, white scar-like areas, unstructured areas with peripheral collections of gray-blue/purple granules, and degenerative changes with blue-gray granules in the marginal area.

Definition

Regression pattern consists of a melanocytic lesion with a white scar-like depigmentation (lighter than the surrounding skin) and/or speckled multiple blue-gray to purple granules (melanophages).

Occurrence

Regression pattern occurs as malignant melanomas, dysplastic nevi, persistent nevi, and occasionally within benign nevi.

Surface Microscopy

There are white scar-like areas (whiter than the surrounding skin) which may be associated with milky red, red-blue, or aggregated blue-gray granules (melanophages; Fig. 164). The blue-gray granules (multiple blue-gray dots) are arranged mainly in the marginal area of whitish degenerative changes. In most lesions there are pigment network fragments, branched streaks, or aggregated globules at the periphery.

Histopathology

There is variable, usually irregularly distributed fibrosis, melanin incontinence, and dilated capillaries within a thickened papillary dermis. The inflammatory cells infiltrate the tumor nests, which are eventually replaced by fibrosis associated with sparse lymphocytic infiltrates.

References

26; 142; 278; 323

Regression Structures

▶ Regression pattern.

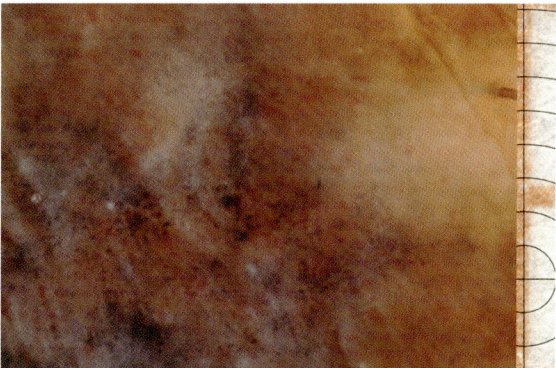

Fig. 164 The boxed-in area of a superficial spreading melanoma (Clark level III, Breslow thickness 0.55 mm) illustrated by regression structures (white scar-like areas and blue-gray pepper-like granules)

Regressive Areas

▶ Regression pattern.

Rete Ridges

Synonyms
Synonyms for rete ridges are stratum malpighii, malpighian stratum, and malpighian rete.

Definition
The living layer of the epidermis, comprising the basal layer, the spinous layer and the granular layer, interdigitates with the dermal papillae. The dermoscopic honeycomb-like reticulation (network) in normal well-pigmented skin and in melanocytic lesions correlates with the rete ridges (Fig. 165). The ridges on the palms and soles correspond to the crista superficialis and the furrows represent the sulcus superficialis.

References
160; 170

Retention Hyperkeratosis

▶ Hyperkeratosis.

Reticular Network

▶ Reticular pattern.

Reticular Pattern

Synonyms
Synonyms for reticular pattern are typical pigment network, reticular network, and honeycomb-like network.

Definition
A reticular pattern is a pigmented network that covers most parts of a melanocytic lesion.

Occurrence
Reticular pattern is the most common pattern in melanocytic lesions.

Surface Microscopy
In benign melanocytic lesions, the pigment network is usually delicate and regular with circular or oval meshes and thins out at the peripheral edge of the lesion (Fig. 166). In dysplastic nevi or melanoma, the network is prominent and irregular, and has an abrupt cut-off at the periphery.

Reference
82

Reticular–Homogeneous Pattern

Definition
Reticular–homogeneous pattern is a melanocytic lesion that represents a pigmented reticular basic pattern that suggests benign alteration (Fig. 167). Other typical features and criteria for melanocytic changes,

☐ **Fig. 165** Double-lined rete ridges of intense sun-induced pigmentation (dorsum) in a 37-year-old woman

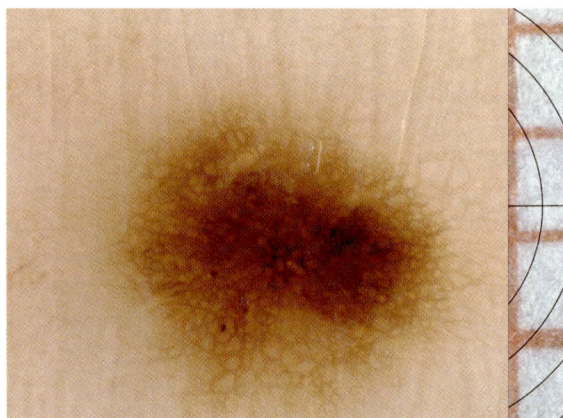

☐ **Fig. 166** Early junctional nevus (jentigo) demonstrates a delicate and regular reticular pattern

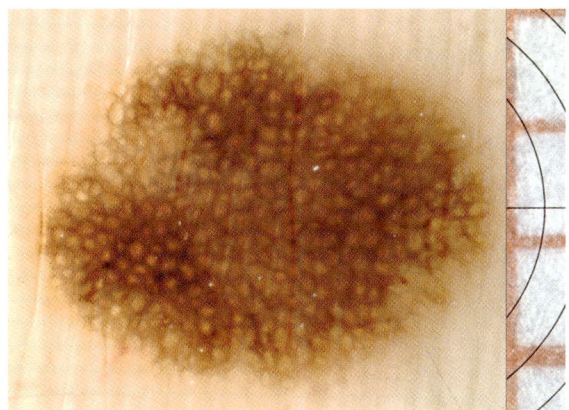

■ **Fig. 167** Combination of a junctional nevus with a lentigo ("jentigo") on the back shows a reticular–homogeneous basic pattern

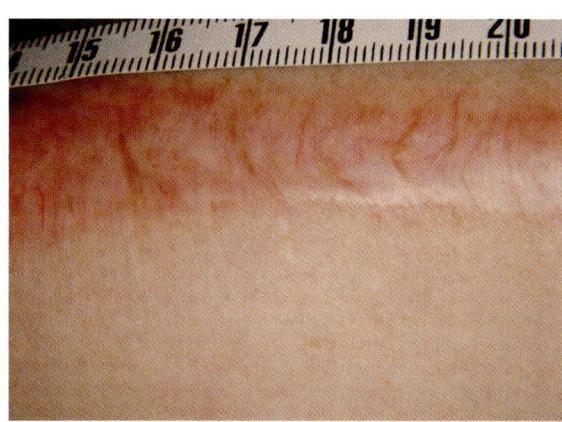

■ **Fig. 168** Vessels of the rope-ladder type in a scar, already visible with the naked eye

e.g., aggregated globules, branched streaks, and dots, are absent.

Reticulo-globular Pattern

▶ Diffuse network with central globules.

Rhexis Bleeding

▶ Nailfold capillaries, alterations.

Rhomboidal Structures

▶ Annular–granular pattern.

Rope–Ladder Pattern

Definition
In long-standing scars, vessels merge across the cleft perpendicularly, generating the appearance of a rope ladder (Fig. 168).

Reference
160

Rosacea-like Dermatitis

▶ Corticosteroid side effects.

Ruby Spot

▶ Hemangioma senile.

Saccular Pattern

Synonym

The synonym for saccular pattern is milky-red globules. Some authors call it "globules."

Definition

Saccular pattern consists of clusters of round, ovoid, polygonal, and spherical reddish, red-blue, red/light-brown, and blue-gray discs up to 0.45 mm in diameter, surrounded by whitish-opaque septa. Some authors use the term "saccular pattern" to describe the base structure of hemangiomas that consist of convoluted capillaries (of the subpapillary plexus) or cavernous large vascular spaces lined with endothelium are seen within the upper dermis and/or subcutis. The tumors often contain mixed elements of capillary and cavernous sinuses.

Occurrence

Saccular pattern occurs as malignant melanomas (specificity >90% and sensitivity >20% for invasive melanomas) and malignant melanoma metastases.

Surface Microscopy

Surface microscopy shows round, ovoid, or polygonal sac-like structures (filled with corpuscular elements, e.g., melanoma cells) that have ill-defined or "hazy" margins and homogeneous coloration. There are several combinations of shading: red-blue; red/light brown; reddish-brownish gray; blue-gray; and dark-brown to black (Figs. 169–172). The redder the sacculi, the more intense the neovascularization. An intraepidermal density of brown granules (melanin) may partially obscure the underlying structures. Most saccular shapes are surrounded by whitish-opaque septa due to the space-occupying process of prolifer-

ating atypical melanocytes, compressing the papillary connective tissue (associated with inflammatory reactive fibrosis) against the rete ridges.

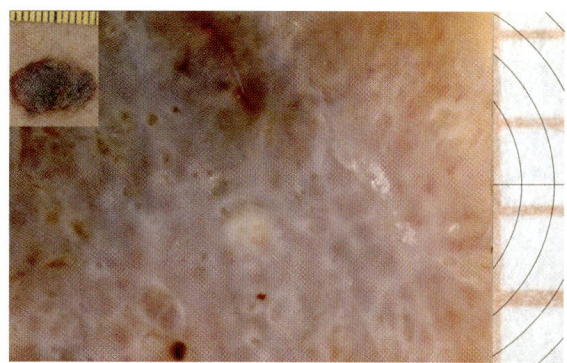

◘ **Fig. 169** Superficial spreading melanoma (Clark Level IV, Breslow thickness 1.15 mm) shows a reddish-brownish gray saccular pattern with whitish-opaque septa

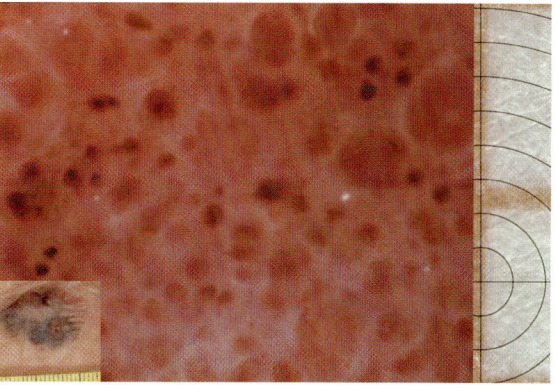

◘ **Fig. 170** Acrolentiginous melanoma (Clark Level V, Breslow thickness 3.1 mm) shows a red-light brown saccular pattern with whitish-opaque septa

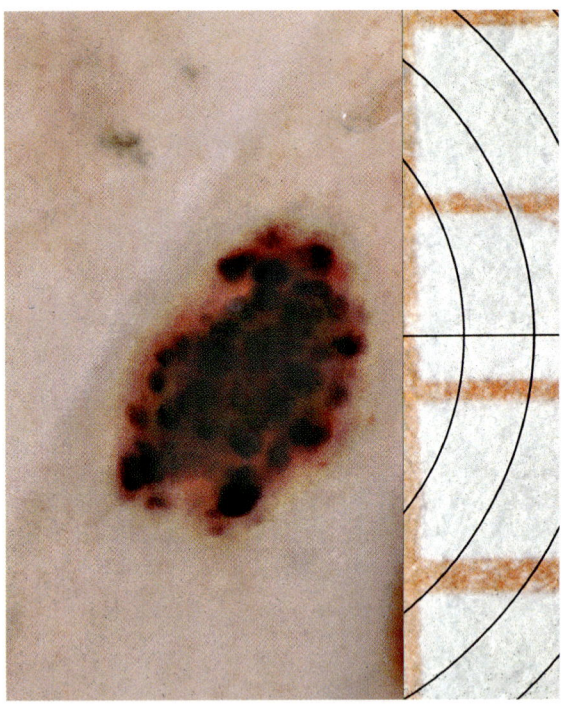

Fig. 171 Malignant melanoma in-transit metastasis of the upper leg shows a dark blue-gray spherical (globular) saccular pattern (atypical melanocytes filling out the whole dermal papillae)

Histopathology

Histopathology shows that the sacculi are round or ovoid junctional nests of proliferating atypical melanocytes. They produce a degree of melanin pigment extension different from that of the epidermal layers. Other features, such as a lymphoid infiltrate, fibrosis, dilated vessels, and neovascularization in the superficial and papillary dermis, are often present.

References

143; 184; 252; 262

Satellitosis

▶ Malignant melanoma metastases, cutaneous.

Scabies

Surface Microscopy

The biting apparatus of Sarcoptes scabiei mites and the two front pairs of legs consist of thick dark-brown chitin layers. In low magnification they take the shape of a dark triangle (hang glider sign). The rear section of the trunk has a brownish hue with light-brown dots, but it is usually poorly visible. The female mite is 0.3×0.4 mm in size. The mites' subcorneal burrows contain eggs and feces (Fig. 173).

References

17; 60; 311

Scar-like Depigmentation

Synonym

The synonym for scar-like depigmentation is white structureless areas.

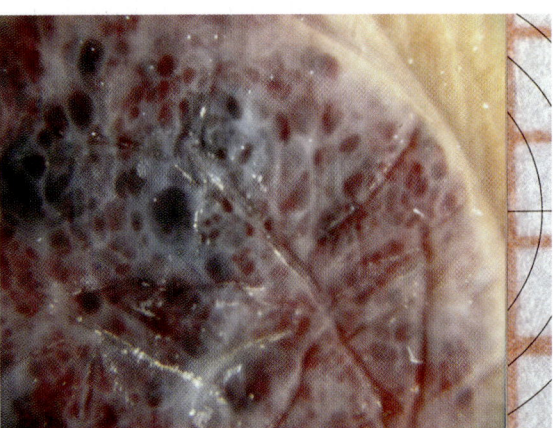

Fig. 172 Hemangioma cavernosum on the thigh demonstrates multiple well-demarcated blue-red to dark-blue lacunae ("saccular pattern") that are tightly clustered and partly separated by whitish-opaque septa

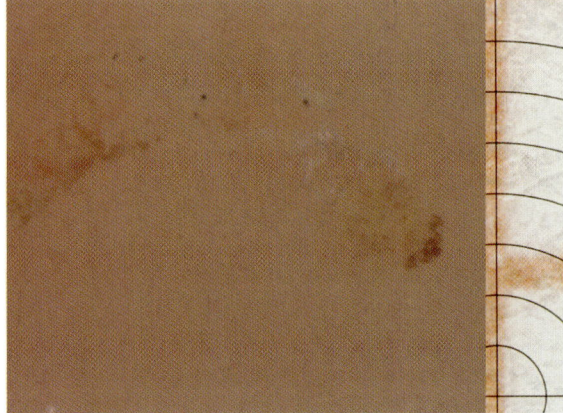

Fig. 173 Sarcoptes scabiei mite, eggs, and feces within the burrow in the stratum corneum

Definition

Scar-like depigmentation consists of irregularly depigmented lesions in the chronic phase of regression which presents as whitish, irregular extensions without any structures (lighter than the surrounding skin; Fig. 174).

Occurrence

Scar-like depigmentation occurs as invasive malignant melanomas (with a specificity of 93% and a sensitivity of 36%), lentigo maligna melanomas, dysplastic nevi, persistent nevi, occasionally within benign nevi, and hemangiomas (presence of multiple red-blue lacunes, absence of any trace of a pigment network).

Surface Microscopy

Whitish reticular extensions may spread throughout the entire lesion.

References

189; 298

Scleroderma

▶ Nail fold capillaries, alterations.

Scleroderma Pattern

Definition

Scleroderma pattern shows changes of the nailfold in scleroderma, representing the triad of diminished cap-

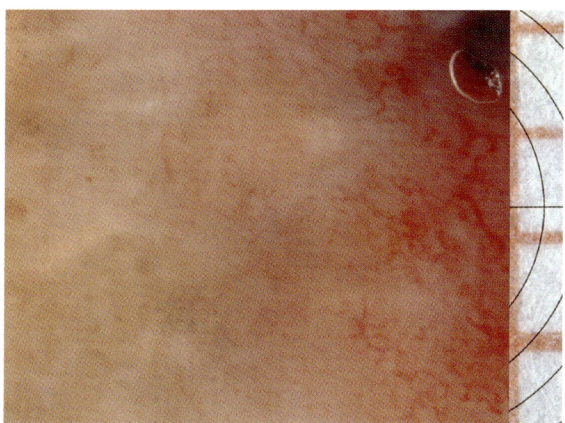

◘ **Fig. 174** Superficial spreading melanoma (Clark level IV, Breslow thickness 1.8 mm) on the upper arm. Scar-like areas of white irregular extensions correspond to zones of regression

illaries, thin loops, intermingled megacapillaries, and pearly shining sclerosis.

References

48; 161

Sebaceous Gland Follicle

The holocrine sebaceous glands follicles are characteristic of human beings and not present in animals. Sebaceous glands open into the hair follicles and secrete an oily semifluid, sebum. Increased amounts of sebum form a huge yellowish brown follicular plug and opening up to 0.4 mm in diameter. Under surface microscopy the follicular channel is surrounded by target-like rims which correspond to the opaque inner-root sheath (i.e., granular layer), the outer-root sheath (i.e., spinous layer), and at the periphery, the more or less pigmented basal lamina. An accumulation of keratinized material, in addition to excessive production of sebum, may form microcomedones. Unlike a normal targetoid sebaceous follicle with a small plug in the center and a relatively broad target-like pattern, the large channel containing a microcomedo (>0.4 mm in diameter) is surrounded by very narrow rims of follicular keratosis.

Sebaceous Gland Hyperplasia

▶ Crown vessels.

Sebaceous Hyperplasia

▶ Crown vessels.

Seborrheic Keratoses

Synonyms

Synonyms for seborrheic keratosis are seborrheic wart, seborrheic verruca, age spot, verruca seborrhoica senilis, and basal cell papilloma.

Definition

Seborrheic keratoses are benign proliferations of keratinocytes within the stratum spinosum (acanthosis) and the basal layer. They are evenly pigmented light- to dark-brown oval macules with sharply demarcated borders and with flat (smooth surface), hyperkeratotic, or warty surface. The macular lesions usually have an endophytic (reticular) growth pattern.

Surface Microscopy

Early lesions often have a finger-printing or network-like pattern (mimicking melanocytic networks; Fig. 175) with sharply demarcated scalloped borders ("moth-eaten") and the jelly sign. An opaque yellowish-brown to gray-brown color can be seen in the lesion. The peripheral follicular rim may be intensely pigmented. Pseudohorncysts are less common within the flat endophytic flat reticular (adenoid) type (Fig. 176). As

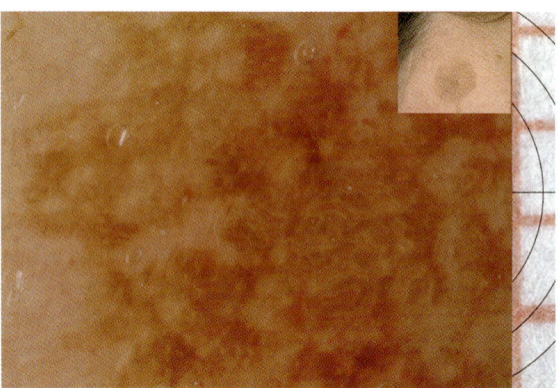

Fig. 175 Partially flat (*left portion*) and partially hyperkeratotic (*central portion*) seborrheic keratosis on the preauricular region characterized by a finger-printing (*left portion*) and a cerebriform (fissures and ridges in the center) pattern. Note the pseudonetwork of facial skin

a seborrheic keratosis becomes more thickened, there may be comedo-like openings (pseudofollicular openings), milia-like cysts (horny pseudocysts), fissures, and ridges (gyri and sulci, cerebriform pattern). In irritated and regressing lesions hairpin-like-shaped blood vessels surrounded by slate-gray granules (melanophages; Fig. 177), diffuse multiple blue-gray dots, or a so-called annular–granular pattern can be found (e.g., lichen-planus-like keratosis which represents regressing seborrheic keratosis or solar lentigo).

Histopathology

Flat (reticular) seborrheic keratoses are characterized by a net-like endophytic (gland-like, i.e., adenoid) or downward growth pattern with hyperplasia of monotonous, slightly basaloid keratinocytes which extend into the superficial dermis. At the basal and suprabasal levels there is an increase of intracellular melanin pigmentation. Pseudohorncysts are not as frequent in the flat types than in the exophytic keratotic–acanthotic or papillomatous types. Some of the variants are deeply pigmented (melanoacanthoma) or can be entirely devoid of pigmentation. Irritated seborrheic keratoses show pseudosquamous eddies (incomplete horn pearls) and inflammatory cells (lymphocytes, neutrophils) in addition to the standard features. The benign lichenoid keratosis is an irritated, often pigmented flat seborrheic keratosis with a band-like inflammatory (lichenoid) dermal infiltrate.

References
22; 53; 83; 93; 288; 298; 316

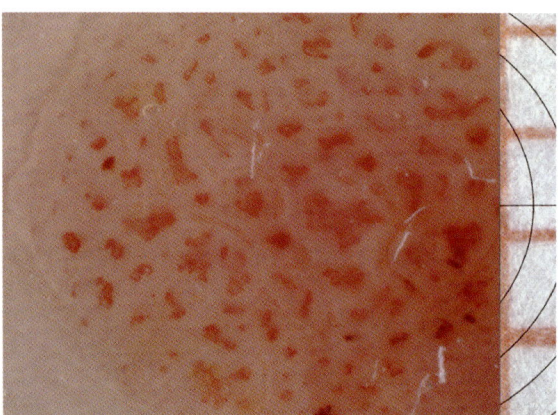

Fig. 176 Acanthotic seborrheic keratosis, devoid of pigmentation and pseudocysts, shows ectatic vessels within the center of hypertrophic dermal papillae

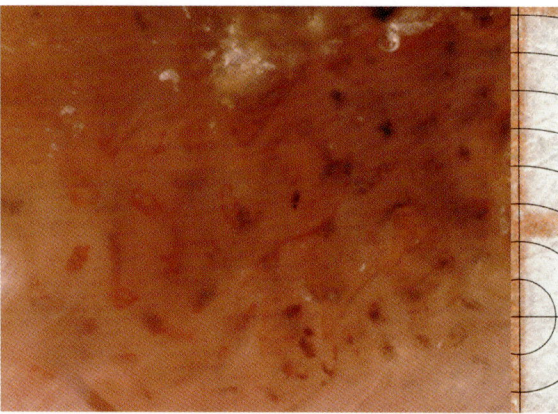

Fig. 177 Irritated seborrheic keratosis with multiple hairpin-like-shaped vessels surrounded by aggregates of blue-gray dots (melanophages)

Seborrheic Verruca

▶ Seborrheic keratoses.

Seborrheic Wart

▶ Seborrheic keratoses.

Segmental Lentiginosis

▶ Nevus spilus.

Senile Lentigo

▶ Solar lentigo.

Sensitivity

Sensitivity is the proportion of a single dermoscopic feature that reveals a positive test result for the feature that the test is intended to identify, for instance, a true-positive feature in malignant melanomas in relation to the same feature of non-melanoma melanocytic nevi, expressed as a percentage.

Septa

▶ Whitish or bluish opaque septa.

Seven-point Checklist

Definition
The seven-point checklist is a diagnostic algorithm that provides a quantitative scoring system for the dermoscopic differentiation between benign melanocytic lesions and melanoma (Table 14).

Reference
26

Single Color

Definition
This represents a single color (brown, black, gray, blue, red, tan) of a pigmented skin lesion.

Surface Microscopy
In melanocytic lesions melanin pigment occupies a varied depth in the skin, from the stratum corneum where it is seen as black; the mid-epidermis, as dark brown; the dermoepidermal junction, as tan; the upper dermis, as gray; and the mid-dermis, as blue.

Reference
189

◘ Table 14 Seven-point checklist. A minimal total score of 3 is required for the diagnosis of melanoma. A total score of < 3 is indicative of non-melanoma. (Modified from [26])

Dermoscopic criterion	Definition	Score
Major criteria		
Atypical pigment network	Black, brown, or gray network with irregular holes and thick lines	2
Blue-white veil	Irregular, structureless area of confluent blue pigmentation with an overlying white "ground-glass" film. The pigmentation cannot occupy the entire lesion and usually corresponds to a clinically elevated part of the lesion	2
Atypical vascular pattern	Linear–irregular or dotted vessels not clearly seen within regression structures	2
Minor criteria		
Irregular streaks	Brown to black, bulbous or finger-like projections irregularly distributed at the edge of a lesion. They may arise from network structures but more commonly do not	1
Irregular dots/ globules	Black, brown, round-to-oval variously sized structures irregularly distributed within the lesion	1
Irregular blotches black	Brown and/or gray structureless areas asymmetrically distributed within the lesion	1
Regression structures	White scare-like depigmentation and/or blue pepper-like granules usually corresponding to a clinically flat part of the lesion	1

Skin of the Palms and Soles

► Normal skin.
► Parallel furrow pattern.

Slate-gray Dots or Granules

► Multiple blue-gray dots.

Slate-gray Ovoid or Larger Areas

► Gray-black and blue-gray ovoid nests.

Slate-gray Pseudopods

► Pseudopods.

Slate-gray Remnants of a Network

► Blue-gray or slate-gray reticular pattern.

Slate-gray Reticular Pattern

► Blue-gray or slate-gray reticular pattern.

Small-diameter Melanocytic Lesions, Differential Diagnosis

Definition

When presented in a dermatological practice, nearly 20% of the malignant melanomas are small-diameter melanomas (<6 mm in maximal diameter). The technique of epiluminescence microscopy (dermoscopy) allows the identification of such melanomas that cannot be discerned by the naked eye or by a pocket lens (Table 15).

References

41; 50; 56; 57; 123; 132; 155; 167; 202; 210; 228; 248; 249; 250; 260; 263; 273; 283; 285; 291; 292; 294; 295; 319

Table 15 Four-step procedure for the differential diagnosis of small-diameter (>6 mm) melanocytic lesions (including malignant melanoma metastases)

Step 1 (suggest benign lesion)	Step 2 (benign/malignant, two features)
Basic pattern	Abrupt cut-off of the trabeculae
Zonal architecture (targetoid)	Peripheral brown/black dots
Cockade architecture	Perivascular melanophages
Radial symmetrical streaks (starburst)	Negative (inverse) network
Central papillary globules in the center of the lesion (target globules)	Brown/black dots on a blue/gray background
Rim of globules at the periphery of the lesion	Regression pattern with blue-gray granules (melanophages)
Slate-gray or brown-black pseudopods with a uniform circumferential position	

Step 3 (mainly malignant)	Step 4 (suggest melanoma)
At least two features of step 2	At least two features of step 3
Peripheral erythema of ectatic vessels (red corona)	Blue-white veil
Grayish patches (irregularly localized)	Slate-gray remnants of a network
Pseudopods	Whitish or bluish opaque septa
Area of target globules (asymmetrically distributed)	Microscopic ovoid blood lakes (microhemorrhages)
Perifollicular circular gray-blue/gray-black pigmentation	
Radial streaming	Polymorphic angiectatic base pattern
Blue-in-pink area	Area of polymorphic vessels
Pseudotrabeculae of melanophages (facial regions)	Saccular pattern (blue-gray, red-light brown)
Trabeculae of melanophages (irregularly distributed)	Gray streaks surrounding the lesion (melanoma cell infarct)
Plaster of Paris-like lacunae	

Solar Lentigo

Synonyms

Synonyms for solar lentigo are senile lentigo, lentigo senilis, "ink-spot" lentigo (a variant), sunburn lentigo, liver spot, and old-age spot.

Definition

Solar lentigo are sharply circumscribed, uniformly light- to dark-brown or black pigmented round-to-oval macules on chronically sun-damaged skin. They consist of melanin-pigmented keratinocytes. Sometimes there are an increased number of large monomorphous melanocytes confined to the basal layer, but not above it. In contrast to freckles, solar lentigines persist when the sun exposure is reduced. In time, some of the solar lentigines evolve into reticulated seborrheic keratoses, whereas other simple lentigines may become junctional nevi.

Surface Microscopy

The lesions often show partially demarcated and irregular, scalloped margins (moth-eaten-like). There may be a faint and irregular network pattern or light-brown structureless areas within the lesion. In some lesions, the network lines are loose and linearly striated (finger-print-like structures; Fig. 178) or the rete ridges can produce grouped circular shapes resembling grape-like clusters. Most of the actinic-damaged and degenerated rete ridges have lost their double-contoured lines. They are narrow and intensely pigmented, often creating a garland-like network of abruptly disrupted pigmentation. The architecture may be similar to that of a reticular seborrheic keratosis. On the scalp and face pseudonetworks are often present. The ink-spot lentigo has an irregularly bordered jet-black pigmented network with thick lines and a highly irregular grid pattern over the entire lesion and ends abruptly at the edge. Brown globules are usually absent, and the vascular pattern is usually prominent.

Histopathology

There is club-shaped elongation of the rete ridges, hyperplasia (increase in the number) of keratinocytes, usually a normal number of melanocytes, and an increased deposition of melanin in the basal keratinocytes. Sometimes there are large melanocytes that are monomorphous, equidistant from one another and unassociated with nests of melanocytes. Solar elastosis is present in the papillary dermis, with or without incontinence of pigment (melanophages).

References

5; 49; 118; 186; 245; 316; 323

Soyer Sign

► Leaf-like areas (Fig. 179).

Specificity

Definition

Specificity is the condition of having a fixed relation to a definite result, i.e., the number of scored negatives for a single feature divided by the total number of lesions without that diagnosis, expressed as a percentage. For

Fig. 178 Solar lentigo on the forehead with a "moth-eaten" edge and "finger-print" pattern

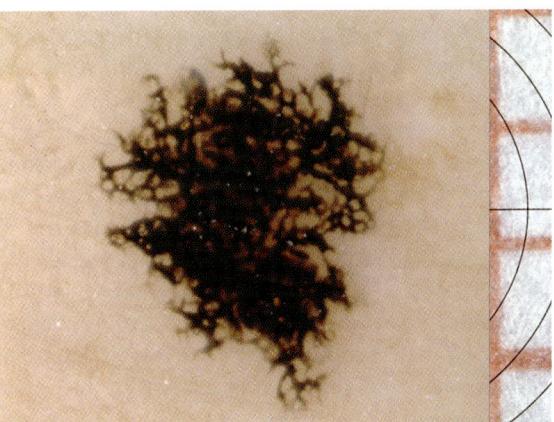

Fig. 179 So-called ink-spot lentigo on the scapular region demonstrates a very prominent network pattern with black network lines and abrupt breaks at the edge

example, percentage of an absent dermoscopic feature in a group of non-melanoma melanocytic lesions in relation to the malignant group of melanocytic lesions.

Spindle Cell Nevus

► Spitz nevus.

Spinous Layer

► Stratum spinosum.

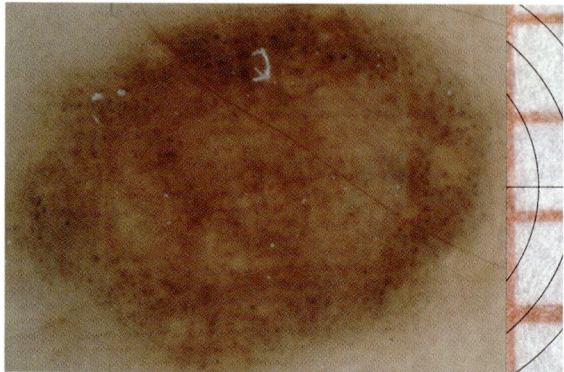

Fig. 180 Spitz nevus with targetoid and symmetrically arranged brown-gray dots and granules on the back in a 20-year-old woman

Spitz Nevus

Synonyms

Synonyms of Spitz nevus are spindle cell nevus, epithelioid cell nevus, Reed nevus (heavily pigmented spindle cell type), and benign juvenile melanoma (obsolete).

Definition

Spitz nevus is a melanocytic nevus that consists of round-to-oval, sharply demarcated papules, most commonly seen in the first and second decades of life. There is a striking variability in size (0.5–2 cm in diameter), form, and color (yellowish-brown, reddish-brown, black or brown).

Surface Microscopy

A variety of patterns can be observed, which are correlated with the cell type and the degree of pigmentation within the lesion. One of the patterns is characterized by regular prominent dark-brown to black network usually forming a characteristic symmetrical corona-like or targetoid pigment structure. A starburst pattern is almost exclusively found in Reed nevi (over 50%). Regular streaks surrounding the lesion symmetrically as well as central blotches or targetoid arranged globules and dots (some with a coffee-bean-like appearance; Figs. 180, 181) are frequently seen. A deep rim of symmetrically distributed globules or pseudopods are often observed at the periphery. Sometimes there are gray-bluish to brown pigmentation or retiform depigmentation in the center. A base pattern which consists of numerous regular dot-like vessels within the center of the papillae is often found in epithelioid cell types. Globules can be a rare sole feature, present in the center or at the periphery. An inverse (negative) pigment

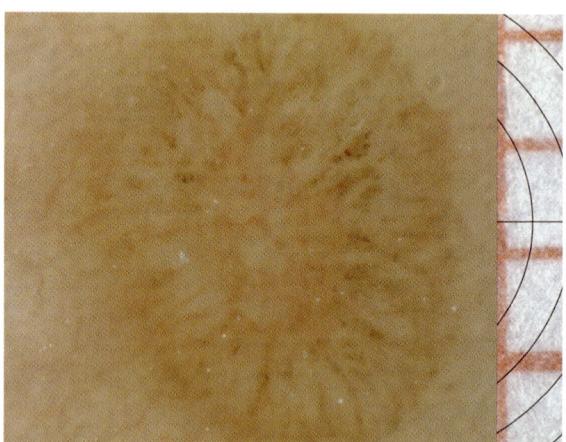

Fig. 181 Targetoid pattern of a Spitz nevus with symmetrically arranged streaks in a radial fashion on the thorax of a 8-year-old boy

network, characterized by dark holes (melanocytic nests in the junctional zone overlaying the tip of the dermal papillae; Fig. 182) and light webs, is a typical basic pattern of some Spitz nevi.

Histopathology

There is usually epidermal change with hypergranulosis, acanthosis, an admixture of epithelioid cells, spindle-shaped cells, multinucleated melanocytes in elongated nests arranged vertically, and clefts between elongated nests and surrounding keratinocytes. The silhouette is symmetric and sharply circumscribed.

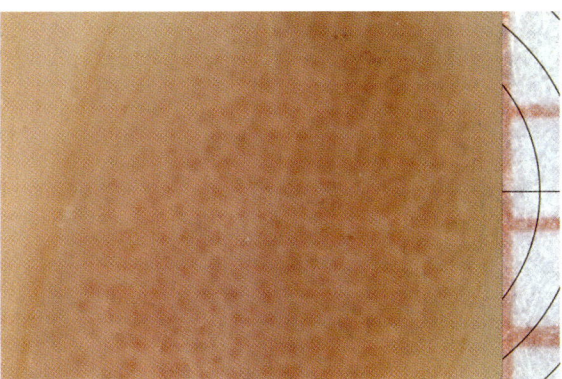

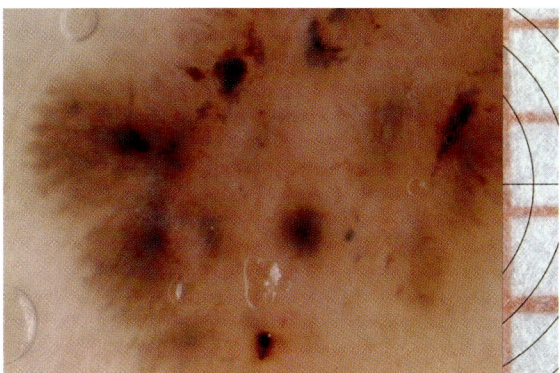

Fig. 182 Spitz nevus shows a regular inverse pigment network with reddish-brown pigmented holes (melanocytic nests in the junctional zone and pinpoint vessels in the center of the dermal papillae) on the thigh of a 44-year-old man

Fig. 183 Pigmented basal cell carcinoma shows spoke-wheel-like structures

References
142; 187; 218; 280; 298

Squamous Cell Carcinoma

Synonyms
Synonyms for squamous cell carcinoma are spinocellular carcinoma and epithelioma spinocellulare.

Definition
Squamous cell carcinoma is a malignant proliferation of squamous cells derived from stratified squamous epithelium or the follicular epithelium of the epidermis. After a variable time period, the tumor cells may grow in a destructive way and invasive tumors can develop.

Surface Microscopy
Surface microscopy shows tumors with a high degree of differentiation (grade I according to Broder) which develop multiple round-to-oval yellowish-brown keratinized areas (subcorneally localized squamous eddies) surrounded by a whitish halo (viable keratinocytes; Fig. 184). Dilated reticular linear vessels surrounding the keratinized structures, as well as polymorphous capillaries with varying calibers and aneurysms, spread throughout the entire lesion. Most malignant neocapillaries are not anatomically associated with the dermal papillae. Microscopic ovoid blood lakes, which represent microhemorrhages next to aneurysmatic vessels, are often seen. Thromboses and sequestrations of capillary loops followed by a so-called Ehring's rhexis bleeding (brown structureless blots in the horny layer)

Isolated, partly atypical and pleomorphic melanocytes may be found in the upper layers of the epidermis. Mitosis can be present. The cells have different levels of pigmentation, prominent nucleoli, mature only minimally in the deeper regions, and are interspersed between bundles of collagen fibers. Dull pink eosinophilic globules (Kamino bodies) are scattered within the proliferating melanocytes and are highly suggestive of the diagnosis.

References
4; 5; 8; 34; 47; 82; 118; 169; 214; 215; 235; 286; 298

Spoke-wheel-like Structures

Synonym
The synonym for spoke-wheel-like structures is Rabinovitz sign.

Definition
These lesions are pigmented with well-defined tan to gray-blue-brown radial projections which meet at an often darker-brown central axis.

Occurrence
These lesions occur as basal cell carcinoma with a high specificity (absence of a pigment network).

Histopathology
Histopathology shows nests of basal cell carcinoma radiating from a follicular epithelium (Fig. 183).

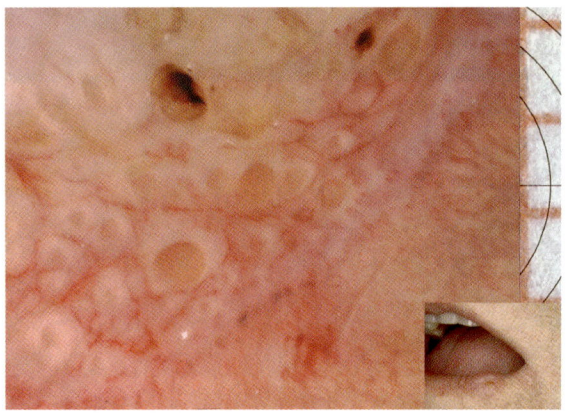

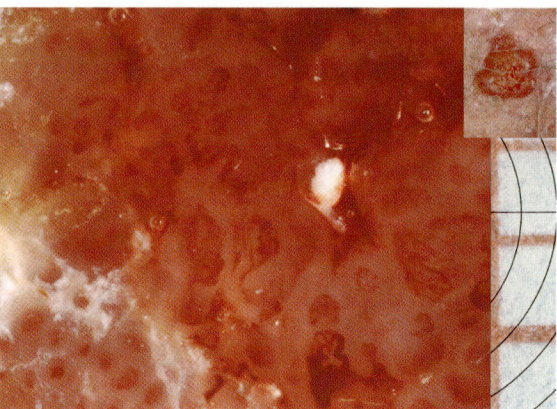

Fig. 184 Highly differentiated squamous cell carcinoma on the lower (pT1a, Broder's grade I) lip shows multiple round-to-oval keratinized areas with whitish halos, irregular vasculature, and the so-called rhexis bleeding

Fig. 185 Dedifferentiated squamous cell carcinoma on the temporal region (pT2c, Broder's grade IV) shows a vascular base pattern which consists of large tortuous, partially bleeding vessels and ectatic capillary loops in the center of the papillae

are typical phenomenons of many well-differentiated tumors (Fig. 185). The more undifferentiated the cells, the more neovascularization can be seen. In less differentiated tumors, the keratinization is less evident. Tumor-associated inflammation may stimulate melanocytes to produce increased melanin (pigment incontinence). Whitish-opaque plaques, which relate to dyskeratoses, are asymmetrically distributed and often near the edge of the lesion. In advanced tumors connective tissue may replace (replacement fibrosis) involution of malignant cells (white structureless scar-like areas).

Histopathology

The atypical keratinocytes, with varying degrees of differentiation, infiltrate into the dermis and may cause local tissue destruction and metastasis. These cells tend to keratinize in forming concentrically layered horn pearls (squamous eddies) beneath the surface. The extent of keratinization correlates with the squamous differentiation within the tumor. A variable rate of mitotic activity is present. A perineural invasion is a poor prognostic parameter. There is marked stromal reaction with an infiltrate of histiocytes, mast cells, lymphocytes, and plasma cells.

References

58; 89; 197; 198; 262; 284

Squamous Cell Carcinoma in Situ

▶ Bowen's disease.

Starburst Pattern

Synonym

The synonym for starburst pattern is radial symmetrical streaks.

Definition

Starburst pattern is a melanocytic lesion with pigmented streaks in a radial arrangement toward the periphery, and a dark or light center is possible.

Occurrence

Starburst pattern is seen mainly in Spitz/Reed nevi (over 50%).

Surface Microscopy

At the periphery one observes homogeneously distributed streaks, pseudopods, or globules (Fig. 186). The surrounding skin can be reddish in color. The center may be homogeneously colored gray-blue to brown-black pigment.

Histopathology

Fascicles and nests of heavily pigmented spindle cells with sharp demarcation at edges are arranged at the dermoepidermal junction and/or papillary dermis. Numerous melanophages are present.

References

20; 47; 82; 279; 298; 301; 314

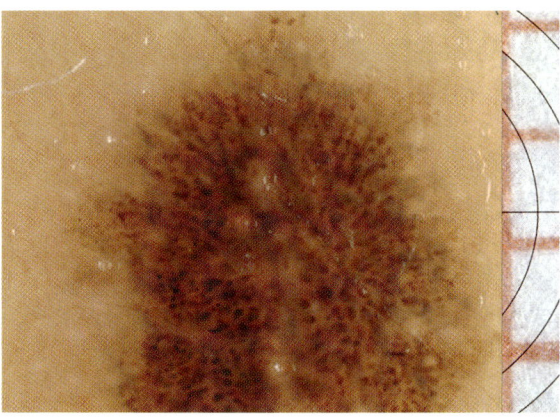

Fig. 186 Spitz nevus in the scapular region demonstrates a starburst pattern

Steel-blue Areas

Definition

Steel-blue areas are homogeneous blue areas devoid of structural components or areas with individual blue globules or dots.

Occurrence

Steel-blue areas occur as blue nevi, combined blue nevi (melanocytic nevus in association with blue nevus), and cutaneous melanoma metastases.

Histopathology

Histopathology shows spindle-shaped, fibroblast-like, or dendritic melanocytes, and numerous melanophages

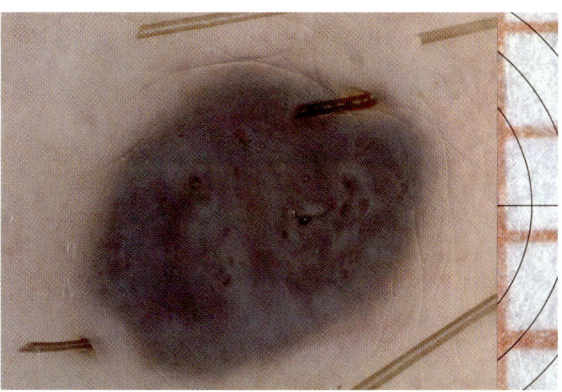

◘ **Fig. 187** Blue nevus on the sternal region represents a steel-blue area

are distributed between the collagen fibers in the dermis (Fig. 187). In cellular blue nevi nests and strands of both spindle and oval epithelioid melanocytes extend into the subcutis.

References

118; 298

Stratum Basale

Synonyms

Synonyms for stratum basale are basal layer, germinative layer, and palisade layer.

Definition

The stratum basale is the deepest layer of the epidermis, one cell thick, composed of dividing stem cells and anchoring cells along the basement membrane.

Stratum Corneum

Synonyms

Synonyms for stratum corneum are scaly or horny layer and corneal layer of epidermis.

Definition

Stratum corneum is the outer layer of the epidermis and consists of approximately 20 cell layers of non-nucleated corneocytes on the trunk or more than 200 on the palms and soles. The scaly layer is an effective epidermal barrier, regulating water loss and allowing selective movement of materials across the skin.

Surface Microscopy

The scaly layer, devoid of blood and melanin, appears yellowish.

Reference

118

Stratum Granulosum

Synonym

The synonym for stratum granulosum is granular layer.

Definition

Stratum granulosum consists of one to three slightly flattened cell layers which contain thick basophilic granules of keratohyalin and lying just above the stratum spinosum and deep into the stratum corneum.

Surface Microscopy

Under surface microscopy a thickening of the granular layer (hypergranulosis) causes a whitish-opaque hue.

Stratum Malpighii

▶ Rete ridges.

Stratum Papillare

Synonyms

Synonyms for stratum papillare are papillary dermis, papillary layer, and corpus papillare.

Definition

Stratum papillare is the upper superficial layer of the corium whose papillae (dermal papillae) interdigitate with the epidermal rete ridges. It contains fine elastin and collagen fibers. The elastic fibers form a fine ramifying network, the subepidermal elastic plexus.

Stratum Reticulare

Synonyms

Synonyms for stratum reticulare are stratum reticulare corii, reticular layer, reticulare cutis, and tunica propria corii.

Definition

Stratum reticulare is the thicker deeper layer of the corium underneath the papillary dermis and consists of dense irregularly arranged connective tissue (network of collagen, reticulin and elastic fibers, fibroblasts, and a mucopolysaccharide ground-substance matrix). It has larger fiber bundles and provides the bulk of the dermis. The cutaneous adnexa in the reticular dermis, including the pilosebaceous units, nails, as well as the eccrine and apocrine sweat glands, are surrounded by a fine fiber network. Actinic atrophy of the skin is caused by regressive changes which involve thinning of the dermis and loss of appendages. The blood vessels are discernible through the translucent skin. Degenerative change of elastic connective tissue fibers causes elastosis.

Surface Microscopy

On surface microscopy the finding of depigmentation may indicate histopathological atrophy, replacement fibrosis, and regression (fibrosis, regression pattern).

Stratum Spinosum

Synonyms

Synonyms for stratum spinosum are spinous layer and prickle cell layer.

Definition

Stratum spinosum is the epidermal layer of polyhedral keratinocytes that are arranged in a horizontal fashion. Shrinkage artifacts and adhesion of these cells at their desmosomal junctions gives a spiny or prickly appearance.

Surface Microscopy

On surface microscopy the thickening of the stratum spinosum (acanthosis) may cause a whitish-yellowish to gray-brownish hue.

Streaks

▶ Radial streaming.

Structureless Areas

Definition

Structureless areas are pigmented skin lesions without any discernible structures (network, globules, etc.) that represent mainly hypopigmented areas. The areas are usually seen in different shades of brown but can also be white, milky red, or blue-gray (e.g., malignant melanoma).

References

142; 298

Subungual Hemorrhage

▶ Blood spots, nail unit.

Subungual Melanocytic Nevus

▶ Brown background, nail unit.

Subungual Melanoma

▶ Acrolentiginous melanoma.

Sunburn Lentigo

▶ Solar lentigo.

Superficial Spreading Melanoma

Synonym

The synonym for superficial spreading melanoma is pagetoid malignant melanoma.

Definition

Superficial spreading melanoma is a slightly raised, multicolored, highly irregular bordered (polycyclic) and laterally spreading malignant tumor that is characterized by the invasion of neoplastic melanocytes throughout the epidermis and into the dermis (Fig. 188). Many superficial spreading melanomas have a nodular portion.

Surface Microscopy

The lesion manifests multiple features including atypical broadened network, pseudopods, radial streaming, peripheral black dots/globules, multiple brown dots, blue-gray dots (peppering), blue-white veil, multiple colors, negative pigment network, scar-like depigmentation (indicating regression), dotted or linearly irregular vasculature, and milky-red to red-brown globules (indicating neovascularization of cell nests and malignant growth).

Histopathology

Characteristically the large epithelioid melanocytes proliferate singly or in nests throughout the epidermis in a so-called pagetoid spread. The tumor may grow downward into the dermis and can infiltrate the adnexal epithelium. The atypical, partly spindle-shaped cells show varying degrees of pigmentation and mitoses. Areas of regression are distinguished by fibrosis and increased melanophages.

References

118; 190

Supernumerary Nipple

Synonyms

Synonyms for supernumerary nipple are accessory nipple and polythelia.

Definition

Supernumerary nipple represents the rudimentary lactiferous ducts in the mammary line.

Surface Microscopy

The whitish-red to light-brown circular and slightly raised rudimentary ductal structure is surrounded by an areola which consists of a pigment network with more or less pigmented lines (grids) and streaks. The inner ring-like zone of the nipple may consist of a reticular pattern of thin thread-like vessels (Fig. 189).

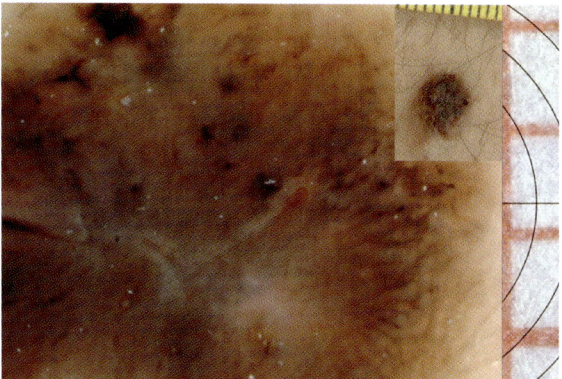

Fig. 188 This multicolored superficial spreading melanoma (Clark level II, Breslow thickness 0.74 mm) has the distinct melanoma features of blue-white veil, peripheral black dots, irregular radial streaming, and an atypical network

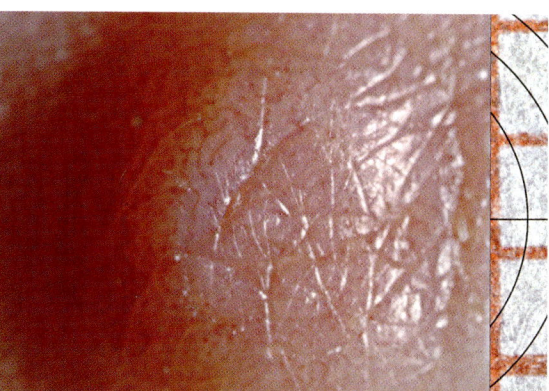

Fig. 189 Supernumerary nipple shows reticular thread-like vessels near the center

Histopathology

The region of the pigmented areola consists of acanthosis with increased basal pigmentation adjacent to lactiferous ducts.

Reference

298

Sutton Nevus

▶ Halo nevus.

Symmetric Pigmentation Pattern

A pigmented skin lesion with symmetry of pattern and texture (not obligatory of shape) along all axes through the center of gravity suggests a benign lesion. When an asymmetric pigmentation pattern lacks symmetry over one or more axes through its center, it is a characteristic feature of nearly all advanced melanomas and atypical/dysplastic melanocytic nevi.

References

188; 204; 205

Tack Phenomenon

Definition

After detaching a lamellar scale from a plaque of a discoid lupus erythematosus plaque, pointed-conical keratotic plugs become visible, originating from the follicle openings (Fig. 190). This typical phenomenon indicates follicular comedo-like hyperkeratosis.

References

13; 37; 58; 61; 329

Target Globules

Synonyms

Synonyms for target globules are area with central papillary globules, area of target globules, mulberry-like structures, and irregular area of slate-gray target globules.

Definition

The globules of melanocytic lesions form target-like architectures or mulberry-like structures.

Occurrence

Target globules occur as benign melanocytic nevi (symmetrically arranged), Clark nevi (symmetrically or asymmetrically arranged), Spitz nevi (symmetrically arranged), papillomatous dermal nevi (symmetrically arranged), and malignant melanomas (asymmetrically arranged).

Surface Microscopy

Globules with a diameter of 0.1–0.4 mm occur in the "holes" of the pigmented network. The color is brown, slate-gray, or black. The spherical aspect is due to a dif-

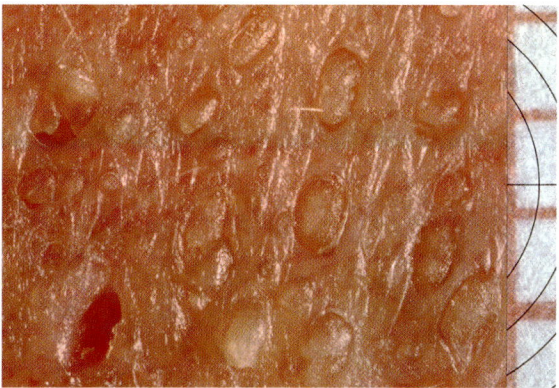

■ **Fig. 190** Discoid lupus erythematosus plaque indicates the tack phenomenon as a result of follicular comedo-like hyperkeratosis. Note the oval hole which was previously filled by a conical keratinized follicular plug

ferent shading, which depends on the localization of the pigment within the dermal papilla. Malignant melanomas or dysplastic nevi may show a mulberry-like arrangement of globules within demarcated and asymmetrically localized zones (Figs. 191, 192).

Histopathology

The globules correspond to aggregations of melanocytes, clumps of melanin, and/or melanophages situated near the top of the dermal papillae and overlying cap-like the central capillary loop.

References

174; 262

Targetoid Pattern

▶ Zonal architecture.

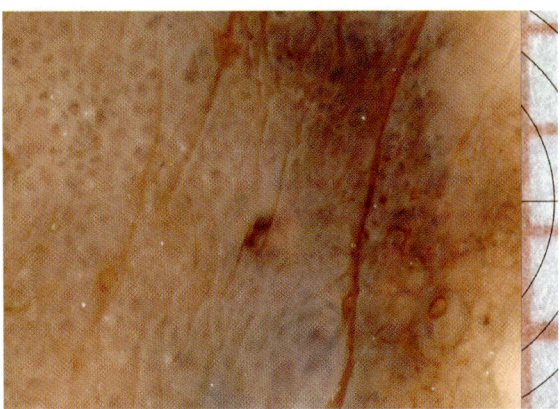

Fig. 191 Unclassified malignant melanoma (Clark level II, Breslow thickness 0.5 mm) in the scapular region shows a mulberry-like arrangement of slate-gray globules near the border of the lesion

Telangiectasia

Synonyms

Synonyms for telangiectasia are angiotelectasia and angiotelectasis.

Definition

Telangiectasia is dilation of the previously existing terminal capillaries and venules in the papillary dermis. Arborizing (tree-like) telangiectases are seen with distinct branching. They occur mainly in basal cell carcinoma and less commonly in invasive melanoma. Regularly distributed loops within hypertrophic papillae are typical feature of seborrheic keratoses.

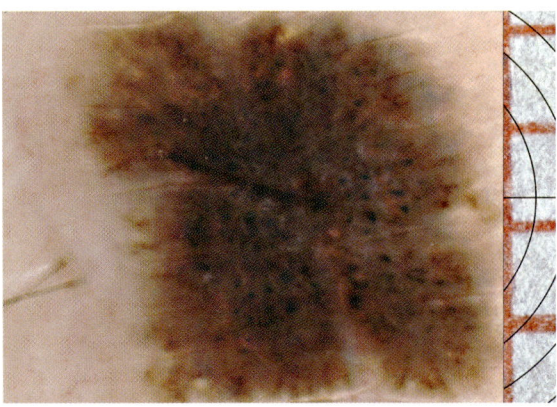

Fig. 192 Spitz nevus in the knee region with a central area of slate-gray target globules

Reference

143

Terminal Hair Follicle

▶ Follicular plug and opening.

Three-point Checklist

Definition

The three-point checklist is a simplified algorithm for the evaluation of pigmented skin lesions (Table 16).

References

130; 173

Total Dermoscopy Score

▶ ABCD rule of dermoscopy.

Trabeculae of Melanophages

Synonyms

Synonyms for trabeculae of melanophages are gray-blue trabecular melanophages and dendritic grayish-blue trabeculae.

Definition

Trabeculae of melanophages are melanocytic lesions that present irregularly distributed trabeculae (streaks)

Table 16 The three-point checklist. (Modified from [173])

Criteria	Definition
Asymmetry	Asymmetric distribution of colors and dermoscopic structures
Atypical network	Pigmented network with irregular holes and thick lines
Blue-white structures	Any type of blue and/or white color including white scar-like depigmentation, blue-whitish veil, and blue pepper-like granules (regression structures)

The presence of more than one criterion suggests a suspicious lesion of loosely aggregated melanophages (blue-gray to purplish-gray granules; Fig. 193).

Occurrence

Trabeculae of melanophages occur as malignant melanoma, regressive melanoma, dysplastic nevus, and occasionally within benign regressive nevi.

References

231; 257; 260; 262; 263

Tree-like Branching

▶ Arborizing vessels.

Tree-like Telangiectasis

▶ Arborizing vessels.

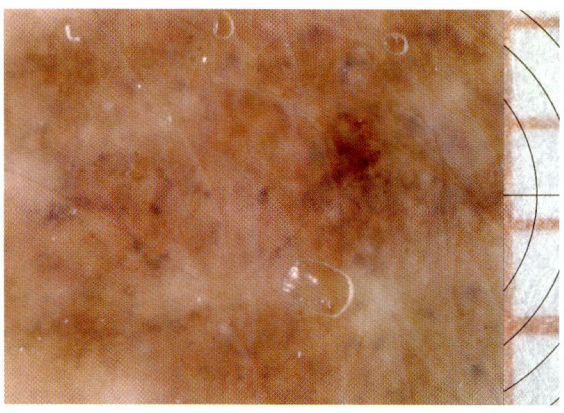

☐ **Fig. 193** Melanoma in situ on the back shows multiple irregularly distributed trabeculae of gray-blue melanophages

Triangular Structure

▶ Scabies.

Unclassified Pattern

Definition

An unclassified pattern is a melanocytic lesion without a typical pattern, e.g., reticular, globular, homogeneous, and definable peripheral or central structures, that suggests dysplastic or malignant changes (Fig. 194). Those changes require either close follow-up or excision.

Unna's Nevus

► Papillomatous or dome-shaped nevus.

Unstructured Areas with Peripheral Collections of Gray-blue/Purple Granules

► Regression pattern.

Urticarial Vasculitis

Definition

Urticarial vasculitis is a chronic recurrent urticarial disease that can be classified in the histological investigation as a leukocytoclastic vasculitis.

Surface Microscopy

Erythematous papules within urticarial lesions reveal a net-like pattern of dilated blood vessels of the subepidermal plexus and/or purpuric dots and globules due to erythrocyte diapedesis suggestive of an underlying vasculitis (Fig. 195). Whitish-opaque areas may result from subepidermal edema. The follicular ostia are not altered.

References

309; 311

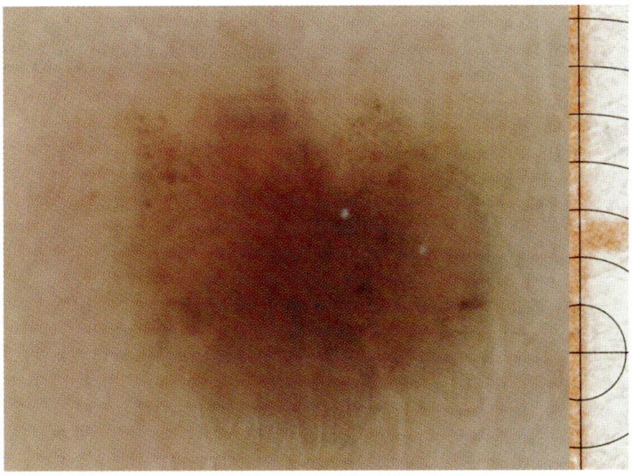

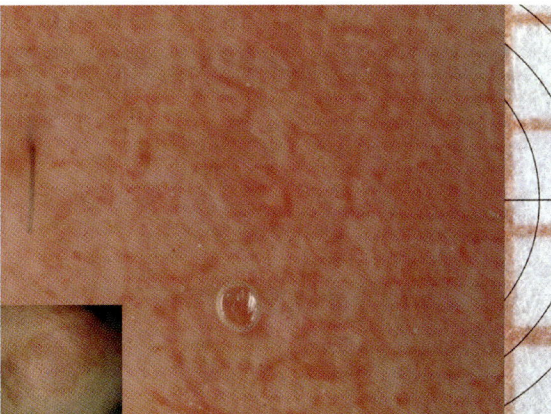

◘ **Fig. 194** Dysplastic junctional nevus on the regio umbilicalis shows an unclassified pattern with irregularly distributed slate-gray globules and dots as well as dilated capillaries of the dermal papillae

◘ **Fig. 195** Urticarial vasculitis on the cheek presents as interfollicular dilated vessels of the subepidermal plexus, purpuric dots, and a light-brown pigmentation of the background (pigment incontinence)

Vascular Lobules

▶ Lacunae.

Vascular Patterns

Definition

A wide variety of vascular structures and patterns exist in the skin, both typical and atypical vascular structures. The most common vascular patterns include: comma-shaped vessels; pin-point vessels; tree-like (arborizing) vessels; hairpin-like-shaped vessels; and radial or wreath-like vessels. Atypical vascular patterns may include linear, dotted, globular, or hairpin-like-shaped red structures irregularly distributed within the lesion, or irregular polymorphous patterns of small vessels running both parallel and vertical to the skin surface. Milky-red or blue-red globules and larger areas reflect vascularized tumor nests. Some of the vascular patterns may be due to neovascularization, and other patterns represent dilated vessels (telangiectasia) in the papillary dermis or red-blue lacunae (lagoons), which correspond to dilated vascular spaces within the papillary dermis.

References

12; 16; 18; 21; 124; 154; 156; 157; 158; 280

Vascular Structures in Skin Tumors

Definition

Vascular structures in skin tumors are various morphological types of vessels associated with various melanocytic and non-melanocytic skin tumors (Table 17).

References

18; 23; 24; 25; 29; 31; 50; 53; 79; 129; 145; 157; 159; 187; 254; 324

Vellus Hair Follicles

Vellus hair follicles are spread over almost the entire body with the exception of the palms, soles, and mucous membranes. The highest density of follicles, ranging from 500 to 850 follicles per square centimeter, is found in facial regions. The diameters of the follicular openings vary between 0.09 and 0.2 mm. Vellus hair follicles produce fine, hardly visible light hair in the center and a small sebaceous gland attached to them.

Surface Microscopy

On surface microscopy, they are seen as well-defined "target" structures. The center of the follicle contains a fine brownish keratin dot (vellus hair) surrounded by the inner-root sheath forming a whitish-opaque rim (i.e., granular layer). A peripherally attaching broader rim corresponds with the more translucent outer-root sheath (i.e., spinous layer). An outermost thinner circle consists of the more or less pigmented basal lamina.

Verruca Seborrhoica Senilis

▶ Seborrheic keratoses.

Vital Histology

▶ In-vivo histology.

◘ **Table 17** Dermoscopic vascular structures of skin tumors. (Adopted from [25])

Vascular structure	Definition
Arborizing vessels	Stem vessels with a large diameter, branching irregularly into the finest terminal capillaries. The vessel is bright red, which is perfectly in focus in the images because of their location on the surface of the tumor (just below the epidermis), e.g., basal cell carcinoma
Dotted vessels	Tiny red dots densely aligned next to each other in a regular fashion, e.g., Spitz nevus. Erythema pinkish color usually seen within areas of regression or at the border of the lesion, e.g., melanoma in situ
Linear–irregular vessels	Linear and irregularly shaped, sized, and distributed red structures, e.g., nodular melanoma
Comma-like-shaped vessels	Coarse vessels that are slightly curved and barely branching, e.g., dermal congenital melanocytic nevus
Polymorphous/atypical	Any combination of two or more different types of vascular structures. The most frequent vessels are the ones which occur between linear–irregular and dotted vessels, e.g., nodular amelanotic part of a melanoma
Hairpin-like-shaped vessels	Vascular loops sometimes twisted and bending, usually surrounded by a whitish halo when seen in keratinizing tumors, e.g., squamous cell carcinoma
Glomerular vessels	Variation on the theme of dotted vessels. They are tortuous capillaries often distributed in clusters, mimicking the glomerular apparatus of the kidney, e.g., Bowen's disease
Milky-red globules/areas	Globules and/or larger areas of fuzzy or unfocused milky-red color usually corresponding to an elevated part of the lesion, e.g., invasive melanoma
Crown vessels	Groups of orderly, bending, scarcely branching vessels located along the border of the lesion, e.g., sebaceous hyperplasia

White and Blue Areas

▶ Regression pattern.

White Scar-like Areas

▶ Regression pattern.

Whitish- or Bluish-Opaque Septa

Definition

The development of opaque septa is due to the space-occupying tumor cell proliferation or blood sinuses juxtaposed to the rete ridges, in addition to an inflammatory reactive fibroplasia.

Occurrence

Opaque septa occur as malignant melanomas and hemangiomas (smooth-bordered red lagoons without either transepidermal melanin output or any trace of pigment network).

Surface Microscopy

In malignant melanomas the septa are associated with the saccular pattern.

Histopathology

Histopathology shows hypergranulosis of the epidermis. Round or oval junctional nests of rapidly proliferating atypical melanocytes within the dermal papillae are separated by whitish-opaque fibrous septa. The walls of dilated blood sinuses compressed to adjacent tissues could also result in similar surface microscopy patterns.

References
262; 263

Wickham's Striation Phenomenon

Especially in aggregated lichen planus papules, there is a fine, milky-white network. It is due to circumscribed thickening of the keratohyalin-containing stratum granulosum (hypergranulosis).

Surface Microscopy

On surface microscopy it creates the typical whitish-opaque hue overlying and sometimes obscuring deeper structures.

Wobble Sign

Definition

Wobble sign comprises the melanocytic nevi which are fleshy or wobble when the dermatoscope is pushed from side to side (e.g., a distinguishing feature of papillomatous nevi, as the keratoses do not wobble).

Reference
51

Zonal Architecture

Synonym

The synonym for zonal architecture is targetoid pattern.

Definition

Zonal architecture is a pigmented lesion that shows different circularly arranged patterns sometimes forming a cockade, e.g., a light center surrounded by a rim of regularly distributed globules and dots or streaks within a light corona at the periphery.

References

260; 263

References

1. Abuzahra F (1996) Die Entwicklung der Auflicht-mikroskopie. Von den experimentellen Anfängen zum Werkzeug der Diagnostik. Waxmann, Münster New York

2. Ackerman AB (1972) Focal acantholytic dyskeratosis. Arch Dermatol 106:702–6

3. Ackerman AB, Mihara I (1985) Dysplasia, dysplastic melanocytes, dysplastic nevi, the dysplastic nevus syndrome, and the relation between dysplastic nevi and malignant melanomas. Hum Pathol 16:87–91

4. Ackerman AB, Maize JC (1987) Pigmented lesions of the skin. Lea and Febiger, Philadelphia

5. Ackerman AB (1990) A dermatopathologist's guide to melanocytic nevi and malignant melanomas for surgeons. In: Conley J (ed) Melanoma of the head and neck. Thieme, Stuttgart New York, pp 9–33

6. Ackerman AB (1993) Dysplastic nevus: rise and fall of a controversial concept. Zentralbl Haut [Suppl] 162:97

7. Ackerman AB (1993) A critique of an N.I.H. consensus development conference about "early" melanoma. Am J Dermatopathol 15:52–8

8. Ackerman AB, Massi D, Nielsen TA (1999) Dysplastic nevus. Atypical mole or typical myth? Ardor Scribendi, Philadelphia

9. Akasu R (1994) Diagnosis and differential diagnosis of malignant melanoma by dermatoscope and videomicroscope. J Dermatol 21:891–3

10. Altmeyer P, Gammal S, Hoffmann K (1990) Blick in die Haut – Ohne Schnitt und Biopsie. Münch Med Wochenschr 18:14–22

11. Altmeyer P (1996) Pitfalls in the diagnosis of pigmented skin tumors. In: Altmeyer P, Hoffmann K, Stücker M (eds) Skin cancer and UV Radiation. Springer, Berlin Heidelberg New York, pp 971–92

12. Altmeyer P, Dirschka T, Hartwig R (1998) Klinikleitfaden Dermatologie. Gustav Fischer, Ulm Stuttgart Jena

13. Altmeyer P, Bacharach-Buhles M (2008) Online–Enzyklopädie der Dermatologie, Venerologie, Allergologie, Umweltmedizin. Springer, Berlin Heidelberg New York

14. Andreassi L, Perotti R, Rubegni P, Burroni M, Cevenini G, Biagioli M, Taddeucci P, Dell'Eva G, Barbini P (1999) Digital dermoscopy analysis for the differentiation of atypical nevi and early melanoma: a new quantitative semiology. Arch Dermatol 135:1459–65

15. Argenyi ZB (1997) Dermoscopy (epiluminescence microscopy) of pigmented skin lesions. Current status and evolving trends. Dermatol Clin 15:79–95

16. Argenziano G, Fabbrocini G, Carli P et al. (1997) Epiluminescence microscopy: criteria of cutaneous melanoma progression. J Am Acad Dermatol 37:68–74

17. Argenziano G, Fabbrocini G, Delfino M (1997) Epiluminescence microscopy. A new approach to in vivo detection of Sarcoptes scabiei. Arch Dermatol 133:751–3

18. Argenziano G, Fabbrocini G, Carli P et al. (1999) Clinical and dermatoscopic criteria for the preoperative evaluation of cutaneous melanoma thickness. J Am Acad Dermatol 40:61–8

19. Argenziano G, Fabbrocini G, Carli P, De Giorgi V, Sammarco E, Delfino M (1998) Epiluminescence microscopy for the diagnosis of doubtful melanocytic skin lesions: comparison of the ABCD rule of dermatoscopy and a new 7-point checklist based on pattern analysis. Arch Dermatol 134:1563–70

20. Argenziano G, Scalvenci M, Staibano S et al. (1999) Dermatoscopic pitfalls in differentiating

pigmented Spitz naevi from cutaneous melanomas. Br J Dermatol 141:788–93

21. Argenziano G, Soyer HP, De Giorgi V, Piccolo D (2000) Dermoscopy: a tutorial. EDRA, 1st edn., Milan

22. Argenziano G, Soyer HP, De Giorgi V, Piccolo D (2000) Dermoscopy: an interactive atlas. EDRA, Milan

23. Argenziano G, Soyer HP (2001) Dermoscopy of pigmented skin lesions: a valuable tool for early diagnosis of melanoma. Lancet Oncol 2:443–9

24. Argenziano G, Soyer HP, Chimenti S et al. (2003) Dermoscopy of pigmented skin lesions: results of a consensus meeting via the Internet. J Am Acad Dermatol 48:679–93

25. Argenziano G, Zalaudek I, Corona R, Sera F, Cicale L, Petrillo G, Ruocco E, Hoffmann-Wellenhof R, Soyer P (2004) Vascular structures in skin tumors. Arch Dermatol 140:1485–9

26. Argenziano G (2005) The seven-point checklist. In: Marghoob AA, Braun RP, Kopf AW (eds) Atlas of dermoscopy. Taylor and Francis, London New York, pp 110–7

27. Arndt KA (1987) Lichen planus. In: Fitzpatrick TB, Eisen AZ, Wolff K et al. (eds) Dermatology in general medicine, 3rd edn. McGraw-Hill, New York, pp 967–73

28. Ascierto PA, Satriano RA, Palmieri G, Parasole R, Bosco L, Castello G (1998) Epiluminescence microscopy as a useful approach in the early diagnosis of cutaneous malignant melanoma. Melanoma Res 8:529–37

29. Bafounta ML, Beauchet A, Aegerter P, Salag P (2001) Is dermoscopy (epiluminescence microscopy) useful for the diagnosis of melanoma? Results of a metaanalysis using techniques adapted to the evaluation of diagnostic tests. Arch Dermatol 137:1343–50

30. Bahmer FA, Rohrer C (1985) Ein Beitrag zur Abgrenzung früher maligner Melanome mittels einer einfachen Methode der hochauflösenden Hautoberflächen–Fotographie. Akt Dermatol 11:149–53

31. Bahmer FA, Fritsch P, Kreusch J, Pehamberger H, Rohrer C, Schindera I, Smolle J, Soyer HP, Stolz W (1990) Terminology in surface microscopy. J Am Acad Dermatol 23:1159–62

32. Bahmer FA, Fritsch P, Kreusch J, Pehamberger H, Rohrer C, Schindera I et al. (1990) Terminology in surface microscopy. Consensus meeting of the Committee on Analytical Morphology of the Arbeitsgemeinschaft Dermatologische Forschung, Hamburg, Federal Republic of Germany, 17 November 1989. Hautarzt 41:513–14

33. Balkau D, Gartmann H, Wischer W, Grootens A, Hagemeier HH, Hundeiker M, Suter L (1988) Architectural features in melanocytic lesions with cellular atypia. Dermatologica 177:129–37

34. Barnhill RL, Barnhill MA, Berwick M et al. (1991) The histologic spectrum of pigmented spindle cell nevus: a review of 120 cases with emphasis on atypical variants. Hum Pathol 22:52–8

35. Barnhill R, Mihm M (1993) The histopathology of cutaneous malignant melanoma. Semin Diagn Pathol 10:47–75

36. Barnhill RL, Fitzpatrick TB, Fandrey K, Kenet RO, Mihm MC Jr, Sober AJ (1995) Color atlas and synopsis of pigmented lesions. McGraw-Hill, New York

37. Bauer R, Orfanos CE (1983) Contemporary aspects of lupus erythematosus and its subjects. I. In: Rook AJ, Maibach HI (eds) Recent advances in dermatology. Churchill Livingstone, Edingburgh, pp 213–36

38. Bauer J, Blum A (2005) Dermoscopic features of common melanocytic nevi of the junctional, compound and dermal type. In: Marghoob AA, Braun RP, Kopf AW (eds) Atlas of dermoscopy. Taylor and Francis, London New York, pp 181–7

39. Behrendt H, Korting HC (1990) Klinische Prüfung von erwünschten und unerwünschten Wirkungen topisch applizierter Glikokortikosteroide am Menschen. Hautarzt 41:2–8

40. Benelli C, Roscetti E, Pozzo VD, Gasparini G, Cavicchini S (1999) The dermoscopic versus the clinical diagnosis of melanoma. Eur J Dermatol 9:470–6

41. Bergman R, Katz I, Lichtig C, Ben-Arieh Y, Moscona AR, Friedman-Birnbaum R (1992) Malignant melanomas with histologic diameters less than 6 mm. J Am Acad Dermatol 26:462–6

42. Binder M, Kittler H, Steiner A, Dawid M, Pehamberger H, Wolff K (1999) Reevaluation of the ABCD rule for epiluminescence microscopy. J Am Acad Dermatol 40:171–6

43. Binder M, Kittler H, Seeber A, Steiner H, Pehamberger H, Wolff K (1998) Epiluminescence microscopy-based classification of pigmented skin lesions using computerised image analysis and an artificial neural network. Melanoma Res 8:261–6

44. Binder M, Braun RP (2005) Principles of dermoscopy. In: Marghoob AA, Braun RP, Kopf AW

(eds) Atlas of dermoscopy. Taylor and Francis, London New York, pp 7–12

45. Blum A, Rassner G, Garbe C (2003) Modified ABC-point-list of Dermatoscopy: a simplified and highly accurate dermatoscopic algorithm for the diagnosis of cutaneous melanocytic lesions. J Am Acad Dermatol 48:672–8

46. Blum A, Luedtke H, Ellwanger U, Rassner G, Garbe C (2005) ABC-point-list of dermoscopy. In: Marghoob AA, Braun RP, Kopf AW (eds) Atlas of dermoscopy. Taylor and Francis, London New York, pp 128–33

47. Blum A, Metzler G, Braun RP, Marghoob AA, Bauer J (2005) Spitz and Reed nevi. In: Marghoob AA, Braun RP, Kopf AW (eds) Atlas of dermoscopy. Taylor and Francis, London New York, pp 195–203

48. Bollinger A, Jäger K, Siegenthaler W (1986) Microangiopathy of progressive systemic sclerosis. Evaluation by dynamic fluorescence videomicroscopy. Arch Intern Med 146:1541–5

49. Bologna J (1992) Reticulated black solar lentigo (ink spot lentigo). Arch Dermatol 128:934–40

50. Bono A, Bartoli C, Moglia D, Maurichi A, Camerini T, Grassi G, Tragni G, Cascinelli N (1999) Small melanomas: a clinical study on 270 consecutive cases of cutaneous melanoma. Melanoma Res 9:583–6

51. Braun RP, Krischer J, Saurat JH (2000) The "wobble sign" in epiluminescence microscopy as a novel clue to the differential diagnosis of pigmented skin lesions. Arch Dermatol 136:940–2

52. Braun RP, Calza AM, Krischer J et al. (2001) The use of digital dermoscopy for the follow-up of congenital nevi: a pilot study. Pediatr Dermatol 18:277–81

53. Braun RP, Rabinovitz H, Oliviero M, Kopf AW, Saurat JH (2002) Dermoscopic diagnosis of seborrheic keratosis. Clin Dermatol 20:270–2

54. Braun RP, Rabinovitz H, Krischer J et al. (2002) Dermoscopy of pigmented seborrheic keratosis. Arch Dermatol 138:1556–60

55. Braun RP, Rabinovitz H, Oliviero M et al. (2002) Dermatoscopie des lésions pigmentées. Ann Dermatol Venerol 129:187–202

56. Braun RP, Saurat JH (2005) Differential dianosis of pigmented lesions of the skin. In: Marghoob AA, Braun RP, Kopf AW (eds) Atlas of dermoscopy. Taylor and Francis, London New York, pp 43–54

57. Braun-Falco O, Stolz W, Bilek P, Merkle T, Landthaler M (1990) Das Dermatoskop. Hautarzt 41:131–6

58. Braun-Falco O, Plewig G, Wolff HH, Winkelmann RK (1991) Dermatology. Springer, Berlin Heidelberg New York

59. Breitbart EW, Hicks R, Kimmig W, Brockmann W, Mohr P (1992) Ultraschall in der Dermatologie. Derm A-Med, Kreuzlingen, Germany

60. Brunetti B, Vitiello A, Delfino S, Sammarco E (1998) Findings in vivo of Sarcoptes scabiei with incident light microscopy. Eur J Dermatol 8:266–7

61. Callen JP (1982) Chronic cutaneous lupus erythematosus. Arch Dermatol 118:412–16

62. Carli P, De Giorgi V, Cattaneo A, Gianotti B (1996) Mucosal melanosis clinically mimicking malignant melanoma: non-invasive analysis by epiluminescence microscopy. Eur J Dermatol 6:434–6

63. Carli P, De Giorgi V, Soyer HP et al. (2000) Dermatoscopy in the diagnosis of pigmented skin lesions: a new semiology for the dermatologist. J Eur Acad Dermatol Venerol 14:353–69

64. Carli P, De Giorgi V, Massi D, Gianotti B (2000) The role of pattern analysis and the ABCD rule of dermoscopy in the detection of histological atypia in melanocytic nevi. Br J Dermatol 143:290–7

65. Carli P, de Giorgi V, Soyer HP, Stante M, Mannone F, Giannotti B (2000) Dermoscopy in the diagnosis of pigmented skin lesions: a new semiology for the dermatologist. J Eur Acad Dermatol Venereol 14:353–69

66. Carrol DM, Billingsley EM, Helm KF (1998) Diagnosing basal cell carcinoma by dermoscopy. J Cutan Med Surg 3:62–7

67. Cascinelli N, Ferrario M, Tonelli T, Leo E (1987) A possible new tool for clinical diagnosis of melanoma: the computer. J Am Acad Dermatol 16:361–7

68. Chen TC, Kuo T, Chan HL (2000) Dermatofibroma is a clonal proliferative disease. J Cutan Pathol 27:36–9

69. Christofolini M, Bauer P, Boi S, Micciolo R et al. (1997) Diagnosis of cutaneous melanoma: accuracy of a computerized image analysis system. Skin Res Technol 3:23–7

70. Clark WH, Reimer RR, Greene M et al. (1978) Origin of familial malignant melanomas from heritable melanocytic lesions. "The B–K mole syndrome". Arch Dermatol 114:732–8

71. Clark W, Elder DE, Guerry D, Epstein NM, Greene MH, van Horn M (1984) The precursor lesions of superficial spreading and nodular melanoma. Hum Pathol 15:1147–65

72. Cohn BA (2000) From sunlight to actinic keratosis to squamous cell carcinoma. J Am Acad Dermatol 42:143–4

73. Conley J, Lattes R, Orr W (1971) Desmoplastic malignant melanoma (a rare variant of spindle cell melanoma). Cancer 28:914–36

74. Conley J (1990) Melanoma of the head and neck. Thieme, Stuttgart New York

75. Connors RC, Ackerman AB (1976) Histological pseudomalignancies of the skin. Arch Dermatol 112:1767–80

76. Cooper HP (1992) Deep penetrating (plexiform spindle cell) nevus. A frequent participant in combined nevus. J Cutan Pathol 19:172–80

77. Curco N, Jucgla A, Bordas X (1992) Dermatofibroma with spreading satellitosis. J Am Acad Dermatol 27:1017–19

78. Curley RK, Cook MG, Fallowfield ME, Marsden RA (1989) Accuracy in clinically evaluating pigmented lesions. Br Med J 299:16–18

79. Dal Pozzo V, Benelli C (1997) Atlas of dermoscopy. EDRA Medical Publishing and New Media, Milan

80. Dal Pozzo V, Benelli C, Roscetti E (1999) The seven features for melanoma: a new dermoscopic algorithm for diagnosis of malignant melanoma. Eur J Dermatol 9:303–8

81. D'Amico D, Vaccaro M, Guarneri C et al. (2001) Videodermatoscopic approach to porokeratosis of Mibelli: a useful tool for the diagnosis. Acta Derm Venerol 81:431–2

82. Dawid M, Pehamberger H, Braun RP, Rabinovitz H (2005) Pattern analysis. In: Marghoob AA, Braun RP, Kopf AW (eds) Atlas of dermoscopy. Taylor and Francis; London New York, pp 118–27

83. De Giorgi V, Massi D, Stante M et al. (2002) False "melanocytic" parameters shown by pigmented seborrheic keratoses: a finding which is not uncommon in dermoscopy. Dermatol Surg 28:776–9

84. De Giorgi V, Stante M, Massi D et al. (2005) Possible histopathologic correlates of dermoscopic features in pigmented melanocytic lesions identified by means of optical coherence tomography. Exp Dermatol 14:56–9

85. Dummer W, Doehnel KA, Remy W (1993) Videomikroskopie in der Differentialdiagnose von Hauttumoren und Sekundärprävention des malignen Melanoms. Hautarzt 44:772–6

86. DuVivier AWP, Williams HC, Brett JV, Higgins EM (1991) How do malignant melanomas present and does this correlate with the seven-point checklist? Clin Exp Dermatol 16:344–7

87. Egbert B, Kempson R, Sagebiel R (1988) Desmoplastic malignant melanoma. A clinicohistopathologic study of 25 cases. Cancer 62:2033–41

88. Ehring F (1953) Vitalmikroskopische Untersuchung zur Lebensdauer der Epidermis. Vortrag, Rheinisch-Westf Dermatologen, 16./17.05.53, Bonn, Germany

89. Ehring F (1956) Über Mikroblutungen am Nagelwall. Eine vitalhistologische Studie. Habil-Schrift, Universitäts-Hautklinik, Münster

90. Ehring F (1958) Geschichte und Möglichkeiten einer Histologie an der lebenden Haut. Hautarzt 9:1–4

91. Ehring F (1965) Die oberen Hautschichten als Ausscheidungsorgan. Hautarzt 16:219–23

92. Ehring F, Schumann J, Voss W (1977) Vitalmikroskopie im Auflicht. Forschungsberichte des Landes NRW Nr. 2621, Westdeutscher Verlag, Wiesbaden, Germany

93. Elgart GW (2001) Seborrheic keratoses, solar lentigines, and lichenoid keratoses. Dermatoscopic features and correlation to histology and clinical signs. Dermatol Clin 19:347–57

94. Feldmann RJ, Maibach HI (1969) Percutaneous penetration of steroids in man. J Invest Dermatol 52:89–94

95. Feldman R, Fellenz C, Gschnait F (1998) Die ABCD-Regel in der Dermatoskopie: Analyse von 500 melanozytären Läsionen. Hautarzt 49:473–6

96. Ferrari A, Soyer HP, Peris K (2000) Central white scarlike patch: a dermatoscopic clue for the diagnosis of dermatofibroma. J Am Acad Dermatol 43:1123–5

97. Friedman R, Rigel DS, Kopf AW (1985) Early detection of malignant melanoma: the role of physician examination and self-examination of the skin. Cancer CA 35:130–51

98. Fritsch P, Pechlaner R (1981) Differentiation of benign from malignant melanocytic lesions using incident light microscopy. In: Ackerman AB, Mihara I (eds) Pathology of malignant melanoma. Masson, New York, pp 301–12

99. Frosch PJ, Wendt H (1985) Human models for quantification of corticosteroid adverse effects. In: Maibach HI, Lowe NJ (eds) Models in dermatology, vol II. Karger, Basel, pp 5–15

100. Gambichler T, Regeniter P, Bechara FG, Orlikov A, Vasa R, Moussa G, Stücker M, Altmeyer P, Hoffmann K (2007) Characterization of benign and malignant melanocytic skin lesions using optical coherence tomography in vivo. J Am Acad Dermatol 57:629–37

101. Gambichler T, Moussa G, Bahrenberg K, Vogt M, Ermert H, Weyhe D, Altmeyer P, Hoffmann K (2007) Preoperative ultrasonic assessment of thin melanocytic skin lesions using a 100-MHz ultrasound transducer: a comparative study. Dermatol Surg 33:818–24

102. Garbe C, Schaumburg-Lever G (1997) Klinik und Histologie des malignen Melanoms. In: Garbe C, Dummer R, Kaufmann R, Tilgen W (eds) Dermatologische Onkologie. Springer, Berlin Heidelberg New York, pp 247–70

103. Garbe C, Blum A (2003) Von der Dermatoskopie zur digitalen Bildanalyse. In: Blum A, Kreusch JF, Bauer J, Garbe C (eds) Dermatoskopie von Hauttumoren. Sieinkopff, Darmstadt, pp 1–6

104. Gilje O, O'Leary PA, Baldes EJ (1953) Capillary microscopic examination in skin diseases. AMA Arch Derm Syph 68:136–47

105. Glogau RG (2000) The risk of progression to invasive disease. J Am Acad Dermatol 42:23–4

106. Goldman L (1951) Some investigative studies of pigmented nevi with cutaneous microscopy. J Invest Dermatol 16:407–26

107. Grant-Kels JM, Bason ET, Grin CM (1999) The misdiagnosis of malignant melanoma. J Am Acad Dermatol 40:539–48

108. Greene MH, Clark WH Jr, Tucker MA et al. (1985) Acquired precursors of cutaneous malignant melanoma. The familial dysplastic nevus syndrome, N Engl J Med 312:91–7

109. Greene MH (1999) The genetics of hereditary melanoma and nevi: 1998 update. Cancer 86:2464–77

110. Grin CM, Saida T (2005) Pigmented nevi of the palms and soles. In: Marghoob AA, Braun RP, Kopf AW (eds) Atlas of dermoscopy. Taylor and Francis, London New York, pp 271–9

111. Guillod JF, Skaria AM, Salomon D, Saurat JH (1997) Epiluminescence videomicroscopy: black dots and brown globules revisited by stripping the stratum corneum. J Am Acad Dermatol 36:371–7

112. Gutkowicz-Krusin D, Elbaum M, Szwaykowsk P, Kopf AW (1997) Can early malignant melanoma be different from atypical melanocytic nevus by in vivo techniques? Skin Res Technol 3:15–22

113. Haas N, Ernst TM, Stüttgen G (1984) Frühdiagnose und Differenzierung von melanozytären Läsionen durch intravitale Makrophotographie. Akt Dermatol 10:156–8

114. Haas N, Ernst TM (1986) Makrophotographische Korrelate zur Histologie bei Precursor-Naevi und SSM in Anlehnung an das Schema von McGovern. Z Hautkr 61:1535–42

115. Hall P, Cladridge E, Morris Smith J (1995) Computer screening for early detection of melanoma: Is there a future? Br J Dermatol 132:325–38

116. Harvell JD, White WL (1999) Persistent and recurrent blue nevi. Am J Dermatopathol 21:506–17

117. Harvell JD, Bastian BC, LeBoit PE (2002) Persistent (recurrent) Spitz nevi: a histopathologic, immunohistochemical, and molecular pathologic study of 22 cases. Am J Surg Pathol 26:654–61

118. Hölzle E, Kind P, Plewig G, Burgdorf W (1993) Malignant melanoma. Diagnosis and differential diagnosis. Schattauer, Stuttgart New York

119. Hoffmann K, Gambichler T, Rick A, Kreutz M, Anschuetz M, Grünendick T, Orlikov A, Gehlen S, Perotti R, Andreassi L, Newton Bishop J, Césarini JP, Fischer T, Frosch PJ, Lindskov R, Mackie R, Nashan D, Sommer A, Neumann M, Ortonne JP, Bahadoran P, Penas PF, Zoras U, Altmeyer P (2003) Diagnostic and neural analysis of skin cancer (DANAOS). A multicentre study for collection and computer-aided analysis of data from pigmented skin lesions using digital dermoscopy. Br J Dermatol 149:801–9

120. Hoegl L, Stolz W, Braun-Falco O (1993) Historical development of skin surface microscopy. Hautarzt 44:182–5

121. Hoffmann R (2001) TrichoScan: combining epiluminescence microscopy with digital image analysis for the measurement of hair growth in vivo. Eur J Dermatol 11:362–8

122. Hoffmann-Wellenhof, Blum A, Wolf IH, Piccolo D, Kerl H, Garbe C, Soyer HP (2003) Atypische melanozytäre Nävi (Clark-Nävi). In: Blum A, Kreusch JF, Bauer J, Garbe C (eds) Dermatoskopie von Hauttumoren. Steinkopff, Darmstadt, pp 35–9

123. Horsch A, Stolz W, Pompl R, Bunk W, Dersch DR, Graf A, Abmayr W, Brauer W, Morfill G (1997) Digital image analysis for better early recognition of malignant melanomas. 5th Congress of the International Society for Skin Imaging, Wien. Skin Res Technol 3:196

124. Hundeiker M, Brehm K (1971) Hautrelief und Capillararchitektur. Arch Dermatol Forsch 242: 78

125. Hundeiker M (1990) Entwicklung und Früherkennung der malignen Melanome. In: AG für Krebsbekämpfung NRW (ed) Kampf dem Krebs. Schürmann and Klagges, Bochum, pp 37–47

126. Imperial A, Helwig EB (1967) Angiokeratoma. A clinicopathological study. Arch Dermatol 95:166–75

127. Jain S, Allen PW (1989) Desmoplastic malignant melanoma and its variants. Am J Surg Pathol 13:358–73

128. Johr R, Stolz W (1997) Lentigo maligna and lentigo maligna melanoma. J Am Acad Dermatol 37:512

129. Johr R (2002) Pink lesions. Clin Dermatol 20:289–96

130. Johr R, Soyer HP, Argenziano G et al. (2004) Dermoscopy: the essentials. Mosby, Edinburgh

131. Jünger M, Steins A, Schlagenhauff B, Rassner G (1999) The microcirculation of malignant melanoma. Hautarzt 50:848–52

132. Kamino H, Kiryu H, Ratech H (1990) Small malignant melanomas: clinicopathologic correlation and DNA ploidy analysis. J Am Acad Dermatol 22:1032–8

133. Karpati S, Torok E, Kosnai I (1986) Discrete palmar and plantar symptoms in children with dermatitis herpetiformis Duhring. Cutis 37:184–7

134. Kaserer C, Koller J (1991) Epidermotrope Melanommetastasen. In: Waclawiczek HW, Gebhart W, Manfreda D, Schlag P (eds) Das maligne Melanom. Springer, Berlin Heidelberg New York, pp 169–72

135. Katz HI, Posalaky Z, McGinley D (1978) Pigmented penile papules with carcinoma in situ changes. Br J Dermatol 99:155–62

136. Katz B, Rao B, Marghoob AA (2005) Vascular lesions, hemangiomas/ angiokeratomas. In: Marghoob AA, Braun RP, Kopf AW (eds) Atlas of dermoscopy. Taylor and Francis, London New York, pp 72–80

137. Katz B, Rao B, Marghoob AA (2005) Dermatofibroma. In: Marghoob AA, Braun RP, Kopf AW (eds) Atlas of dermoscopy. Taylor and Francis, London New York, pp 81–5

138. Katz B, Rao B (2005) Pigmented actinic keratosis. In: Marghoob AA, Braun RP, Kopf AW (eds) Atlas of dermoscopy. Taylor and Francis, London New York, pp 86–9

139. Katz B, Rao B, Marghoob AA (2005) Blue nevus/ combined nevus. In: Marghoob AA, Braun RP, Kopf AW (eds) Atlas of dermoscopy. Taylor and Francis, London New York, pp 188–94

140. Kawabata Y, Tamaki K (1998) Distinctive dermatoscopic features of acral lentiginous melanoma in situ from plantar melanocytic nevi and their histopathologic correlation. J Cutan Med Surg 2:199–204

141. Kawabata Y, Ohara K, Hino H, Tamaki K (2001) Two kinds of Hutchinson's sign, benign and malignant. J Am Acad Dermatol 44:305–7

142. Kaya G, Braun RP (2005) Histopathological correlation in dermoscopy. In: Marghoob AA, Braun RP, Kopf AW (eds) Atlas of dermoscopy. Taylor and Francis, London New York, pp 23–41

143. Kenet RO, Kang S, Kenet BJ, Fitzpatrick TB, Sober AJ, Barnhill RL (1993) Clinical diagnosis of pigmented lesions using digital epiluminescence microscopy: grading protocol and atlas. Arch Dermatol 129:157–74

144. Kittler H, Seltenheim M, Dawid M et al. (2000) Frequency and characteristics of enlarging common melanocytic nevi. Arch Dermatol 136:316–20

145. Kittler H, Pehamberger H, Wolff K, Binder M (2002) Diagnostic accuracy of dermoscopy. Lancet Oncol 3:159–65

146. Kittler H (2005) Diagnostic accuracy of dermoscopy/dermatoscopy. In: Marghoob AA, Braun RP, Kopf AW (eds) Atlas of dermoscopy. Taylor and Francis, London New York, pp 313–6

147. Klein LJ, Barr RJ (1990) Histologic atypia in clinically benign nevi. A prospective study. J Am Acad Dermatol 22:275–82

148. Kopf AW, Levine LJ, Rigel DS, Friedman RJ, Levenstein M (1985) Prevalence of congenital-nevus-like nevi, nevi spili, and café-au-lait spots. Arch Dermatol 121:766–9

149. Kopf AW, Friedman RJ, Rigel DS (1990) Atypical mole syndrome. J Am Acad Dermatol 22:117–18

150. Kornberg R, Ackerman AB (1975) Pseudomelanoma. Recurrent melanocytic nevus following partial surgical removal. Arch Dermatol 111:1588–90

151. Kornberg R, Harrts M, Ackerman AB (1978) Epidermotropically metastatic malignant melanoma. Arch Derm 114:67–9

152. Kossard S, Doherty E, Murray E (1987) Neurotrophic melanoma. A variant of desmoplastic melanoma. Arch Dermatol 123:907–12

153. Krause W (1995) Videomicroscopy in differential diagnosis of skin tumors and in secondary prevention of malignant melanoma. Hautarzt 46:211

154. Kreusch J, Rassner G (1991) Auflichtmikroskopie pigmentierter Hauttumoren. Thieme, Stuttgart New York

155. Kreusch J (1992) Merkmalsanalyse melanozytischer Hautveränderungen mittels Auflichtmikroskopie. Inaugural Dissertation, Tübingen, Germany

156. Kreusch J, Rassner G, Trahn C, Pietsch-Breitfeld B, Henke D, Selbmann HK (1992) Epiluminescent microscopy: a score of morphological features to identify malignant melanoma. Pigment Cell Res (Suppl 2):295–8

157. Kreusch J, Koch F (1996) Auflichtmikroskopische Charakterisierung von Gefäßmustern in Hauttumoren. Hautarzt 47:264–72

158. Kreusch J, Koch F (1997) Vascular structures are important features for diagnosis of melanoma and other skin tumors by incident light microscopy. Melanoma Res (Suppl 7):38

159. Kreusch J (2002) Vascular patterns in skin tumors. Clin Dermatol 20:248–54

160. Kreusch JF (2005) Diagnosis of amelanotic melanoma by dermoscopy: the importance of vascular structures. In: Marghoob AA, Braun RP, Kopf AW (eds) Atlas of dermoscopy. Taylor and Francis, London New York, pp 246–56

161. Kreusch JF (2005) Nailfold capillaries. In: Marghoob AA, Braun RP, Kopf AW (eds) Atlas of dermoscopy. Taylor and Francis, London New York, pp 307–12

162. Kuhn A, Mahrle G (1992) Problemfälle bei der histologischen Diagnostik melanozytärer Hauttumoren. In: Burg G, Hartmann AA, Konz B (eds) Onkologische Dermatologie. Springer, Berlin Heidelberg New York, pp 85–8

163. Lambert WC, Lapidus A, Rao BK (2001) Melanoma diagnosis by computerized analysis of clinical images. Arch Dermatol 137:377–8

164. Langley RG, Rajadhyaksha M, Dwyer PJ, Sober AJ, Flotte TJ, Anderson RR (2001) Confocal scanning laser microscopy of benign and malignant melanocytic skin lesions in vivo. J Am Acad Dermatol 45:365–76

165. Lorentzen H, Weismann K, Secher L, Petersen CS, Larsen FG (1999) The dermatoscopic ABCD rule does not improve diagnostic accuracy of malignant melanoma. Acta Derm Venerol 79:469–72

166. Lynch HT, Frichot BC III, Lynch JF (1978) Familial atypical multiple mole-melanoma syndrome. J Med Genet 15:352–6

167. MacKie RM (1986) Early recognition of malignant melanoma. J Am Acad Dermatol 15:707–8

168. MacKie RM (1971) An aid to the preoperative assessment of pigmented lesions of the skin. Br J Dermatol 85:232–8

169. Maize JC, Ackerman AB (1987) Pigmented lesions of the skin. Lea and Febiger, Philadelphia

170. Malvehy J, Puig S (2005) Breslow depth prediction by dermoscopy. In: Marghoob AA, Braun RP, Kopf AW (eds) Atlas of dermoscopy. Taylor and Francis, London New York, pp 257–70

171. Marghoob AA, Kopf AW (1997) Persistent nevus: an exception to the ABCD rule of dermoscopy. J Am Acad Dermatol 36:474–5

172. Marghoob AA, Blum R, Nossa R, Busam KJ, Sachs D, Halpern A (2001) Agminated atypical (dysplastic) nevi. Case report and review of the literature. Arch Dermatol 137:917–20

173. Marghoob AA, Fu JM (2005) The ABCD-E scoring system and the three-point checklist. In: Marghoob AA, Braun RP, Kopf AW (eds) Atlas of dermoscopy. Taylor and Francis, London New York, pp 134–9

174. Marghoob AA, Fu JM, Sachs D (2005) Dermoscopic features of congenital melanocytic nevi. In: Marghoob AA, Braun RP, Kopf AW (eds) Atlas of dermoscopy. Taylor and Francis, London New York, pp 141–59

175. Marghoob AA, Korzenko A (2005) Recurrent (persistent) nevi. In: Marghoob AA, Braun RP, Kopf AW (eds) Atlas of dermoscopy. Taylor and Francis, London New York, pp 204–7

176. Marique H, Weinberger AB, LeRoy EL (1982) Early detection of scleroderma spectrum disorders by in vivo capillary microscopy. J Rheumatol 9:289–91

177. Marks R, Wilson-Jones E (1971) Purpura in dermatitis herpetiformis. Br J Dermatol 84:386–8

178. Marks R, Rennie G, Selwood TS (1988) Malignant transformation of solar keratoses to squamous cell carcinoma. Lancet 1:795–7

179. Massi D, De Giorgi V, Carli P, Santucci M (2001) Diagnostic significance of the blue hue in dermoscopy of melanocytic lesions: a dermoscopic–pathologic study. Am J Dermatopathol 23:463–9

180. Massi D, De Giorgi V, Soyer HP (2001) Histopathologic correlates of dermoscopic criteria. Dermatol Clin 19:259–68

181. Mayer J (1997) Systematic review of the diagnostic accuracy of dermatoscopy in detecting malignant melanoma. Med J Aust 167:206–10

182. McGovern VJ (1976) Metastatic melanoma. In: McGovern VJ (ed) Malignant melanoma. Wiley, New York London Sydney Toronto, pp 15–120

183. Menzies SW, Crotty K, McCarthy W (1995) The morphologic criteria of the pseudopod in surface microscopy. Arch Dermatol 131:436–40

184. Menzies SW, Ingvar C, McCarthy WH (1996) A sensitivity and specificity analysis of the surface microscopy features of invasive melanoma. Melanoma Res 6:55–62

185. Menzies SW, Ingvar C, Crotty K, McCarthy WH (1996) Frequency and morphologic characteristics of invasive melanomas lacking specific surface microscopic features. Arch Dermatol 132:1178–82

186. Menzies SW, Crotty KA, Ingvar C, McCarthy WH (1996) An atlas of surface microscopy of pigmented skin lesions. McGraw-Hill, Sydney New York San Francisco

187. Menzies SW, Westerhoff K, Rabinovitz H, Kopf A, McCarthy W, Katz B (2000) The surface microscopy of pigmented basal cell carcinoma. Arch Dermatol 136:1012–16

188. Menzies SW, Crotty KA, Ingvar C, McCarthy WH (2003) An atlas of surface microscopy of pigmented skin lesions. Dermoscopy, 2nd edn. McGraw-Hill, Sydney New York San Francisco

189. Menzies SW (2005) The Menzies method. In: Marhoob AA, Braun RP, Kopf AW (eds) Atlas of dermoscopy. Taylor and Francis, London New York, pp 99–109

190. Menzies SW (2005) Superficial spreading melanoma. In: Marghoob AA, Braun RP, Kopf AW (eds) Atlas of dermoscopy. Taylor and Francis, London New York, pp 209–20

191. Menzies SW (2005) Nodular melanoma. In: Marghoob AA, Braun RP, Kopf AW (eds) Atlas of dermoscopy. Taylor and Francis, London New York, pp 234–8

192. Menzies SW (1999) Automated epiluminescence microscopy: human vs machine in the diagnosis of melanoma. Arch Dermatol 135:1538–40

193. Megahed M, Hofmann U, Flür M, Hölzle E (1993) Das polypoide maligne Melanom. Hautarzt 44:437–9

194. Minkin A, Rabhan MB (1982) Office nailfold capillary microscopy using ophthalmoscope. J Am Acad Dermatol 7:190–3

195. Moncrieff M, Cotton S, Claridge E, Hall P (2002) Spectrophotometric intracutaneous analysis: a new technique for imaging pigmented skin lesions. Br J Dermatol 146:448–57

196. Monticone G, Colonna L, Palermi G, Bono R, Puddu P (2000) Quantitative nailfold capillary microscopy findings in patients with acrocyanosis compared with patients having systemic sclerosis and control subjects. J Am Acad Dermatol 42:787–90

197. Moss R, Stoecker WV, Lin S-J, Muruganandhan S, Chu K-F, Poneleit KM, Mitchell CD (1989) Skin cancer recognition by computer vision. Comput Med Imaging Graph 13:31–6

198. Moy RL (2000) Clinical presentation of actinic keratoses and squamous cell carcinoma. J Am Acad Dermatol 42:8–10

199. Morton C, MacKie RM (1998) Clinical accuracy of the diagnosis of cutaneous malignant melanoma. Br J Dermatol 138:283–7

200. Murali A, Stoecker WV, Moss RH (2000) Detection of solid pigment in dermatoscopy images using texture analysis. 6:193–8

201. Nachbar F, Stolz W, Merkle T, Cognetta AB, Vogt T, Landthaler M, Bilek P, Braun-Falco O, Plewig G (1994) The ABCD rule of dermoscopy. High prospective value in the diagnosis of doubtful melanocytic skin lesions. J Am Acad Dermatol 30:551–9

202. Neuber H, Lippold A, Hundeiker M (1991) Nicht-diagnostizierte maligne Melanome. Hautarzt 42:220–2

203. Niedner R, Johannböcke R (1991) Ausgewählte humanpharmakologische Modelle zur Untersuchung topischer Glukokortikoide. TW Dermatol 21:298–306

204. Nilles M, Kerner K, Weyers W, Schill WB (1991) Malignitätshinweise im dermatoskopischen und auflichtmikroskopischen Bild. Z Hautkr 66: 688–90

205. Nilles M, Boedeker R, Schill W (1994) Surface microscopy of nevi and melanomas: clues to melanoma. Br J Dermatol 130:349–55

206. Novice FM, Collison DW, Burgdorf WHC et al. (1994) Disorders of hyperpigmentation. In: Nov-

ice FM (ed) Handbook of genetic skin disorders. Saunders, Philadelphia, pp 195–8

207. Oguchi S, Saida T, Koganehira Y et al. (1998) Characteristic epiluminescent microscopic features of early malignant melanoma on glabrous skin: a videomicroscopic analysis. Arch Dermatol 134:563–8

208. Pang BK, Kossard S (1992) Surface microscopy in the diagnosis of micropapular cutaneous metastatic melanoma. J Am Acad Dermatol 27:775–6

209. Paschoal FM (1996) Early diagnosis of melanoma by surface microscopy (dermatoscopy). Rev Paul Med 114:1220–1

210. Paul E (1991) Problematik der klinischen und histologischen Einordnung von Frühformen maligner Melanome. In: Meigel W, Lengen W, Schwenzer G (eds) Diagnostik and Therapie maligner Melanome. Diesbach, Berlin, pp 106–19

211. Pehamberger H, Steiner A, Wolff K (1987) In vivo epiluminescence microscopy of pigmented skin lesions. I. Pattern analysis of pigmented skin lesions. J Am Acad Dermatol 17:571–83

212. Pehamberger H, Binder M, Steiner A, Wolff K (1993) Early recognition and prognostic markers of melanoma. Melanoma Res 3:279–84

213. Pehamberger H, Binder M, Steiner A, Wolf K (1993) In vivo epiluminescence microscopy: improvement of early diagnosis of melanoma. J Invest Dermatol 100:356S–62S

214. Pellacani G, Martini M, Seidenari S (1999) Digital videomicroscopy with image analysis and automatic classification of Spitz nevus. Skin Res Technol 5:226–72

215. Pellacani G, Cesinaro AM, Seidenari S (2000) Morphological features of Spitz naevus as observed by digital videomicroscopy. Acta Derm Venerol 80:117–21

216. Pellacani G, Cesinaro AM, Seidenari S (2005) In vivo assessment of melanocytic nests in nevi and melanomas by reflectance confocal microscopy. Mod Pathol 18:469–74

217. Peris K, Altobelli E, Ferrari A et al. (2002) Interobserver agreement on dermatoscopic features of pigmented basal cell carcinoma. Dermatol Surg 28:643–5

218. Polsky D (2005) Pigmented basal cell carcinoma. In: Marghoob AA, Braun RP, Kopf AW (eds) Atlas of dermoscopy. Taylor and Francis, London New York, pp 55–9

219. Pompl R, Bunk W, Horsch A, Abmayr W, Morfill G, Brauer W, Stolz W (1999) Computer vision of melanocytic lesions using MELDOQ. Sixth Congress of the International Society for Skin Imaging, London. Skin Res Technol 5:150

220. Pritchett RM, Pritchett PS (1982) Zosteriform speckled lentiginous nevus with giant melanosomes. Cutis 30:329–34

221. Provost N, Kopf AW, Rabinovitz HS, Oliviero MC, Toussaint S, Kamino HH (1997) Globulelike dermoscopic structures in pigmented seborrheic keratosis. Arch Dermatol 133:540–1

222. Puppin D, Salomon D, Saurat JH (1993) Amplified surface microscopy. Preliminary evaluation of a 400-fold magnification in the surface microscopy of cutaneous melanocytic lesions. J Am Acad Dermatol 28:923–7

223. Rabinovitz H, Kopf A, Katz B (1998) Atlas of dermatoscopy [educational CD-ROM]. MMA Worldwide Group, Miami

224. Rallan D, Bush NL, Bamber JC, Harland CC (2007) Quantitative discrimination of pigmented lesions using three-dimensional high-resolution ultrasound reflex transmission imaging. J Invest Dermatol 127:189–95

225. Rampen F, Rümke P (1988) Referral pattern and accuracy of clinical diagnosis of cutaneous melanoma. Acta Derm Venerol 68:61–4

226. Rand R, Baden HP (1983) Commentary: Darier–White disease. Arch Dermatol 119:81–3

227. Rassner G (1988) Früherkennung des malignen Melanoms. Hautarzt 39:396–401

228. Rassner G, Holzschuh J (1995) Auflichtmikroskopie. In: Plewig G, Korting HC (eds) Fortschritte der praktischen Dermatologie und Venerologie, Band 14. Springer, Berlin Heidelberg New York, pp 241–5

229. Reed RJ, Leonhard DD (1979) Neutrophic melanoma. A variant of desmoplastic melanoma. Am J Surg Pathol 3:301–11

230. Reiman HM, Goellner JR, Woods JE, Mixter RC (1987) Desmoplastic melanoma of the head and neck. Cancer 60:2269–74

231. Rhodes AR (1995) Comment on: "Malignant melanoma in epiluminescent microscopy". In: Sober AJ, Fitzpatrick TB (eds) Yearbook of dermatology 1995. Mosby, St. Louis Baltimore Boston, pp 296–8

232. Rhodes AR (1999) Benign neoplasias and hyperplasias of melanocytes. In: Fitzpatrick's dermatology in general medicine. McGraw-Hill, New York, pp 1037–43

233. Rigel DS (1997) Epiluminescence microscopy in clinical diagnosis of pigmented skin lesions? Lancet 349:1566–7

234. Rongioletti F, Miracco C, Gambini C, Pastorino A, Tosi P, Rebora A (1996) Tumor vascularity as a prognostic indicator in intermediate-thickness (0.75–4 mm) cutaneous melanoma. Am J Dermatopathol 18:474–7

235. Rubegni P, Ferrari A, Cevenini G, Piccolo D, Burroni M, Perotti R, Peris K, Taddeucci P, Biagioli M, Dell'Eva G, Chimenti S, Andreassi L (2001) Differentiation between pigmented Spitz naevus and melanoma by digital dermoscopy and stepwise logistic discriminant analysis. Melanoma Res 11:37–44

236. Rütten A, Goos M (1989) Palmoplantare Purpura bei herpetiformer Dermatitis Duhring. Hautarzt 40:640–3

237. Ryan TJ (1980) Microcirculation in psoriasis: blood vessels, lymphatics, and tissue fluids. Pharmacol Ther 10:27–64

238. Saida T, Oguchi S, Ishihara Y (1995) In vivo observation of magnified features of pigmented lesions on volar skin using videomacroscope: usefulness of epiluminescence technique in clinical diagnosis. Arch Dermatol 131:298–304

239. Saida T, Oguchi S, Miyazaki A (2002) Dermoscopy for acral pigmented skin lesions. Clin Dermatol 20:279–85

240. Saida T, Miyazaki A, Grin CM (2005) Acrolentiginous melanoma. In: Marghoob AA, Braun RP, Kopf AW (eds) Atlas of dermoscopy. Taylor and Francis, London New York, pp 221–33

241. Salasche SJ (2000) Epidemiology of actinic keratoses and squamous cell carcinoma. J Am Acad Dermatol 42:4–7

242. Salopek TG, Kopf AW, Stefanato CM et al. (2001) Differentiation of atypical moles (dysplastic nevi) from early melanomas by dermoscopy. Dermatol Clin 19:337–45

243. Saphier J (1920) Dermatoscopy. Arch Dermatol 128:1–19

244. Sato S, Takehara K, Soma Y, Tsuchida T, Ishibashi Y (1993) Diagnostic significance of nailfold bleeding in scleroderma spectrum disorders. J Am Acad Dermatol 28:198–203

245. Schiffner R, Schiffner-Rohe J, Vogt T, Landthaler M, Wlotzke U, Cognetta A, Stolz W (2000) Improvement of early recognition of lentigo maligna using dermoscopy. J Am Acad Dermatol 42:25–32

246. Schiffner R (2005) Dermoscopy on the face. In: Marghoob AA, Braun RP, Kopf AW (eds) Atlas of dermoscopy. Taylor and Francis, London New York, pp 280–8

247. Schmidt K, Mensing H (1987) Kapillarmikroskopie bei Bindegewebserkrankungen. Hautarzt 38:327–30

248. Schmoeckel C, Wagner-Größer G, Braun-Falco O (1985) Klinische Diagnostik initialer maligner Melanome. Hautarzt 36:558–62

249. Schmoeckel C, Braun-Falco O (1987) Diagnosis of early malignant melanoma: sensitivity and specificity of clinical and histological criteria. Pigment Cell 8:96–106

250. Schmoeckel C (1987) Dysplastische Naevi und Melanomvorläufer. In: Braun-Falco O, Schill WB (eds) Fortschritte der praktischen Dermatologie und Venerologie, Bd 11. Springer, Berlin Heidelberg New York, pp 356–60

251. Schulz C (1996) Gefäßveränderungen melanozytärer Tumore in der Auflichtmikroskopie. Zentralbl Haut 167:594

252. Schulz C, Stücker M, Schulz H, Altmeyer P, Hoffmann K (1999) Correlation between epiluminescence microscopy characteristics of malignant melanomas and Clark's level of invasion. Hautarzt 50:785–90 [in German]

253. Schulz H (1988) Früherkennung kortikosteroidbedingter epidermaler Veränderungen mit der Methode der hochauflösenden Hautoberflächen-Fotografie. Therapiewoche 38:2254–60

254. Schulz H (1992) Angiektatische Strukturelemente benigner und maligner Pigmentzelltumore in der Auflichtmikroskopie. Akt Dermatol 18:295–8

255. Schulz H (1992) Epiluminescent microscopy score for the differential diagnosis of dysplastic nevi]. Hautarzt 43:487–90 [in German]

256. Schulz H, Nietsch KH, Höhler T (1993) Early detection of glucocorticoid-specific epidermal alterations using skin surface microscopy. In: Korting HC, Maibach HI (eds) Topical glucocorticoids with increased benefit/risk ratio. Karger, Basel Freiburg Paris, pp 132–9

257. Schulz H (1994) Malignant melanoma in epiluminescent microscopy. Hautarzt 45:15–19

258. Schulz H (1996) Dysplastic nevi in the differential diagnosis of malignant melanoma using epiluminescence microscopy. Hautarzt 47:109–13

259. Schulz H, Noebel A (1996) Diagnostic problems of desmoplastic melanoma in a boy with xeroderma pigmentosum. Dermatol Surg 22:96–8

260. Schulz H (1997) Epiluminescence microscopic characteristics of small-diameter malignant melanomas. Hautarzt 48:904–9

261. Schulz H (2000) Epiluminescence microscopy features of cutaneous malignant melanoma metastases. Melanoma Res 10:273–80

262. Schulz H (2001) Auflichtmikroskopische Vitalhistologie. Dermatologischer Leitfaden. Springer, Berlin Heidelberg New York

263. Schulz H (2003) Melanommetastasen. In: Blum A, Kreusch JF, Bauer J, Garbe C (eds) Dermatoskopie von Hauttumoren. Steinkopff, Darmstadt, pp 51–6

264. Schumann J (1965) Vitalmikroskopie der Haut mit dem Spaltopakilluminator nach Vonwiller. Leitz–Mitt Wiss Techn 111:119

265. Schumann J (1970) Neue Möglichkeiten in der Technik der Vitalmikroskopie an der Haut. Z Wiss Mikrosk 70:1–10

266. Seidenari S, Pellacani G, Pepe P (1998) Digital videomicroscopy improves diagnostic accuracy for melanoma. J Am Acad Dermatol 39:175–81

267. Seidenari S, Pellacani G (2002) Surface microscopy features of congenital nevi. Clin Dermatol 20:263–7

268. Seidenari S, Martela A, Pellicani G (2003) Polarized light-surface microscopy for description and classification of small and medium-sized congenital melanocytic nevi. Acta Derm Venerol 83:271–6

269. Seidenari S, Pellicani G, Gianetti A (1999) Digital videomicroscopy and image analysis with automatic classification for detection of thin melanomas. Melanoma Res 9:163–71

270. Semmelmeyer U, Burgdorf WHC, Stolz W (2005) The ABCD rule. In: Marghoob AA, Braun RP, Kopf AW (eds) Atlas of dermoscopy. Taylor and Francis, London New York, pp 91–8

271. Semmelmayer U, Burgdorf WHC, Stolz W (2005) Lentigo maligna melanoma. In: Marghoob AA, Braun RP, Kopf AW (eds) Atlas of dermoscopy. Taylor and Francis, London New York, pp 239–54

272. Sexton M, Sexton CW (1991) Recurrent pigmented melanocytic nevus. A benign lesion not to be mistaken for malignant melanoma. Arch Pathol Lab Med 115:122–6

273. Shaw HM, McCarthy WH (1992) Small-diameter malignant melanoma: a common diagnosis of New South Wales, Australia. J Am Acad Dermatol 27:679–82

274. Slade J, Marghoob AA, Salopek TG et al. (1995) Atypical mole syndrome: risk factor for cutaneous malignant melanoma and implications for management. J Am Acad Dermatol 32:479–94

275. Smithers BM, McLeod GR, Little JH (1992) Desmoplastic melanoma: patterns of recurrence. World J Surg 16:186–90

276. Smolle J, Soyer H-P, Hoffmann-Wellenhof R et al. (1989) Vascular architecture of melanocytic skin tumors: a quantitative immunohistochemical study using automated image analysis. Pathol Res Pract 185:740–5

277. Sober AJ, Burstein JM (1994) Computerized digital image analysis: an aid for melanoma diagnosis – preliminary investigations and brief review. J Dermatol 21:885–90

278. Soyer HP, Smolle J, Hödl S et al. (1989) Surface microscopy: a new approach to the diagnosis of cutaneous pigmented tumors. Am J Dermatopathol 11:1–10

279. Soyer HP, Kenet RO, Wolf IH et al. (2000) Clinicopathological correlation of pigmented skin lesions using dermoscopy. Eur J Dermatol 10:22–8

280. Soyer HP, Argenziano G, Chimenti S, Menzies SW, Pehamberger H, Rabinovitz HS, Stolz W, Kopf AW (2001) Dermoscopy of pigmented skin lesions. An atlas based on the Consensus Net Meeting on Dermoscopy 2000. EDRA, Milan

281. Soyer HP, Argenziano G, Chimenti S, Ruocco V (2001) Dermoscopy of pigmented skin lesions. Eur J Dermatol 11:270–6

282. Soyer HP, Argenziano G, Ruocco V, Chimenti S (2001) Dermoscopy of pigmented skin lesions (part II). Eur J Dermatol 11:483–98

283. Stagnelli I, Seidenari S, Serafini M, Pellacani G, Bucchi L (1999) Diagnosis of pigmented skin lesions by epiluminescence microscopy: determinants of accuracy improvement in a nationwide training programme for practical dermatologists. Public Health 113:237–42

284. Stedman's Medical Dictionary (2000) Lippincott Williams and Wilkins, Philadelphia Baltimore New York

285. Steiner A, Pehamberger H, Wolff K (1987) In vivo epiluminescence microscopy of pigmented skin lesions. II. Diagnosis of small pigmented skin lesions and early detection of malignant melanoma. J Am Acad Dermatol 17:584–91

286. Steiner A, Pehamberger H, Binder M, Wolf K (1992) Pigmented Spitz nevi: improvement of the diagnostic accuracy by epiluminescence microscopy. J Am Acad Dermatol 27:697–701

287. Steiner A, Binder M, Schemper M, Wolff K, Pehamberger H (1993) Statistical evaluation of epiluminescence microscopy criteria for melano-

cytic pigmented skin lesions. J Am Acad Dermatol 29:581–8

288. Stern R, Boudreaux C, Arndt KA (1991) Diagnostic accuracy and appropriateness of care for seborrheic keratoses. A pilot study of an approach to quality assurance for cutaneous surgery. J Am Med Assoc 265:74–7

289. Stewart DM, Altman J, Mehregan AH (1978) Speckled lentiginous nevus. Arch Dermatol 114:895–6

290. Stolz W, Schmoeckel C, Landthaler M, Braun-Falco O (1989) Association of early malignant melanoma with nevocytic nevi. Cancer 63:550–5

291. Stolz W, Bilek P, Merkle T, Landthaler M, Braun-Falco O (1991) Verbesserung der klinischen Diagnose von pigmentierten Hautveränderungen in der Kindheit mit dem Dermatoskop. Monatsschr Kinderheilkd 139:110–13

292. Stolz W, Landthaler M (1994) Classification, diagnosis and differential diagnosis of malignant melanoma. Chirurg 65:145–52

293. Stolz W, Riemann A, Cognetta AB, Pillet L, Abmayr W, Hözl D, Bilek P, Nachbar F, Landthaler M, Braun-Falco O (1994) ABCD rule of dermatoscopy: a new practical method for early recognition of malignant melanoma. Eur J Dermatol 4:521–7

294. Stolz W (1996) Computer screening for early detection of melanoma: Is there a future? Br J Dermatol 135:146

295. Stolz W, Schiffner R, Pillet L, Vogt T, Harms H, Schindewolf T, Landthaler M, Abmayr W (1996) Improvement of monitoring of melanocytic skin lesions with the use of computerized acquisition and surveillance unit with a skin surface microscopic television camera. J Am Acad Dermatol 35:202–7

296. Stolz W (1997) Auflichtmikroskopische Diagnose des malignen Melanoms. In: Garbe C, Dummer R, Kaufmann R, Tilgen W (eds) Dermatologische Onkologie. Springer, Berlin Heidelberg New York, pp 281–9

297. Stolz W, Pompl R, Burgdorff T, Horsch A, Bunk W, Schiffner R, Gläßl A, Morfill G, Abmayr W (1998) Computerisierte Verlaufskontrolle und bildanalytische Auswertung pigmentierter Hautveränderungen. Z Dermatol 184:170–5

298. Stolz W, Braun-Falco O, Bilek P, Landthaler M, Burgdorf WHC, Cognetta AB (2002) Color atlas of dermatoscopy. Blackwell, Berlin Vienna

299. Stoughton RB, Cornell RC (1988) Topical coticosteroids in dermatology. In: Christophers E, Schöpf E, Kligman AM, Stoughton RB (eds) Topical corticosteroid therapy. Raven Press, New York, pp 1–12

300. Stücker M, Horstmann I, Röchling A, Hofmann K, Nüchel C, Altmeyer P (1996) Differential diagnosis of skin tumors using tumor microcirculation. In: Altmeyer P, Hoffmann K, Stücker M (eds) Skin cancer and UV radiation. Springer, Berlin Heidelberg New York, pp 999–1006

301. Suster S (1994) Hyalinizing spindle and epithelioid cell nevus. A study of five cases of a distinctive histologic variant of Spitz nevus. Am J Dermatopathol 16:593–8

302. Thomas L, Ronger-Savlé S (2005) Dermoscopic examination of melanonychia striata. In: Marghoob AA, Braun RP, Kopf AW (eds) Atlas of dermoscopy. Taylor and Francis, London New York, pp 289–98

303. Tripp JM, Kopf AW (2005) Dysplastic nevus (atypical mole). In: Marghoob AA, Braun RP, Kopf AW (eds) Atlas of dermoscopy. Taylor and Francis, London New York, pp 160–72

304. Tripp JM, Wang SQ, Polsky D, Kopf AW (2005) Benign patterns of clinically atypical nevi. In: Marghoob AA, Braun RP, Kopf AW (eds) Atlas of dermoscopy. Taylor and Francis, London New York, pp 173–80

305. Tronnier M, Kreusch JF (2003) Fallbeispiele melanozytärer Hautveränderungen. In: Blum A, Kreusch JF, Bauer J, Garbe C (eds) Dermatoskopie von Hauttumoren. Steinkopff, Darmstadt, pp 78–84

306. Vázquez-López F, Alvarez-Cuesta CC, Hildalgo Garcia Y, Pérez Oliva N (2001) The handheld dermatoscope improves the recognition of Wickham striae and capillaries in lichen planus lesions. Arch Dermatol 137:1376

307. Vázquez-López F, Maldonado Seral C, López-Escobar M, Pérez Oliva N (2003) Dermoscopy of pigmented lichen planus lesions. Clin Exp Dermatol 28:554–5

308. Vázquez-López F, Manjón Haces JA, Maldonado Seral C et al. (2003) Dermoscopic features of plaque psoriasis and lichen planus: new observations. Dermatology 207:157–66

309. Vázquez-López F, Maldonado Seral C, Soler Sánchez T et al. (2003) Surface microscopy for discriminating between common urticaria and urticarial vasculitis. Rheumatology 42:1079–82

310. Vázquez-López F, Kreusch J, Marghoob AA (2004) Dermoscopic semiology: further insights into vascular features by screening a large spectrum of nontumoral skin lesions. Br J Dermatol 150:226–31

311. Vázquez-López F, Kreusch JF, Marghoob AA (2005) Other uses of dermoscopy. In: Marghoob AA, Braun RP, Kopf AW (eds) Atlas of dermoscopy. Taylor and Francis, London New York, pp 299–306

312. Wade TR, Kopf AW, Ackerman AB (1979) Bowenoid papulosis of the genitalia. Arch Dermatol 115:306–8

313. Waldmann V (2000) Dermatoscopic diagnosis of malignant melanoma. Acta Derm Venerol 80:223

314. Walsh N, Crotty K, Palmer A et al. (1998) Spitz nevus versus spitzoid malignant melanoma: an evaluation of the current distinguishing histopathologic criteria. Hum Pathol 29:1105–12

315. Wang SQ, Katz B, Rabinovitz H et al. (2000) Lessons on dermoscopy no. 4. Poorly defined pigmented lesion. Diagnosis: pigmented BCC. Dermatol Surg 26:605–6

316. Wang SQ, Rabinovitz H, Oliviero MC (2005) Dermoscopic patterns of solar lentigines and seborrheic keratoses. In: Marghoob AA, Braun RP, Kopf AW (eds) Atlas of dermoscopy. Taylor and Francis, London New York, pp 60–71

317. Weidner F, Altendorf A, Neumüller G (1981) Metastasierungsmuster. In: Weidner F, Tonak J (eds) Das maligne Melanom der Haut. Perimed, Erlangen, pp 75–86

318. Westerhoff K, Menzies S (2003) Pigmentierte Basalzellkarzinome. In: Blum A, Kreusch JF, Bauer J, Garbe C (eds) Dermatoskopie von Hauttumoren. Steinkopff, Darmstadt, pp 57–8

319. Wolf IH, Kerl H, Soyer HP, Binder M, Pehamberger H, Fritsch P, Wolff K (1997) Epilumineszenzmikroskopie bei der Diagnose von pigmentierten Hauttumoren. Hautarzt 48:353–62

320. Wolf IH, Smolle J, Soyer HP, Kerl H (1998) Sensitivity in the clinical diagnosis of malignant melanoma. Melanoma Res 8:425–9

321. Wolff K (1983) Lupus erythematodes: Klinische Variationsbreite und Diagnostik. In: Braun-Falco O, Burg G (eds) Fortschritte der praktischen Dermatologie und Venerologie, Bd 10. Springer, Berlin Heidelberg New York, pp 214–9

322. Wolff K, Binder M, Pehamberger H (1994) Epiluminescence microscopy: a new approach to the early detection of melanoma. Adv Dermatol 9:45–56

323. Yadav S, Vossaert KA, Kopf AW, Silverman M, Grin-Jorgensen C (1993) Histopathologic correlates of structures seen on dermoscopy (epiluminescence microscopy). Am J Dermatopathol 15:297–305

324. Zalaudek I, Argenziano G, Kerl H, Soyer HP, Hoffmann-Wellenhof R (2003) Amelanotic/hypomelanotic melanoma: Is dermatoscopy useful for diagnosis? J Deutsche Dermatol Ges 1:369–73